CARING FOR THE ALZHEIMER PATIENT

GOLDEN AGE SERIES

Including the latest research...

Caring for the
Alzheimer
Patient

THIRD EDITION

A PRACTICAL GUIDE

EDITED BY
RAYE LYNNE DIPPEL, PH.D. AND
J. THOMAS HUTTON, M.D., PH.D.

GOLDEN AGE BOOKS

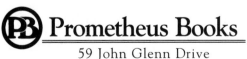 Prometheus Books

59 John Glenn Drive
Amherst, New York 14228-2197

Published 1996 by Prometheus Books

00 99 98   5 4 3 2

Library of Congress Cataloging-in-Publication Data

Caring for the Alzheimer patient : a practical guide / edited by Raye Lynne
    Dippel and J. Thomas Hutton. — 3d ed.
        p.   cm. — (Golden age series)
    Includes bibliographical references
    ISBN 1–57392–108–4 (pbk. : alk. paper)
    1. Alzheimer's disease—Patients—Rehabilitation. 2. Alzheimer's disease—Patients—Care. 3. Alzheimer's disease—Patients—Family relationships. I. Dippel, Raye Lynne. II. Hutton, J. Thomas. III. Series.
RC523.C37   1996
616.8′3103—dc20   96–29306
                                                                                        CIP

Printed in the United States of America on acid-free paper

Contents

7044

6   Caring for the Alzheimer Patient

Preface to the Third Edition

The last few years have brought us much closer to understanding the complicated and often puzzling disease known as Alzheimer's. Unfortunately, this better understanding of the physiological basis of Alzheimer's disease has not led to a cure or significant differences in diagnosis or treatment. This third edition of *Caring for the Alzheimer Patient: A Practical Guide* provides insight into what has been learned the last few years since the second edition was printed, but it also retains the time-tested information for the day-to-day care of the Alzheimer patient, which readers have found quite valuable. Fifteen of the seventeen chapters have been revised to reflect the newest information available to caregivers. It is hoped that this new information, combined with the old, will assist all of those readers who seek to improve their caregiving skills, and ultimately improve the quality of life for those Alzheimer patients under their care.

Raye Lynne Dippel, Ph. D.   J. Thomas Hutton, M.D., Ph.D.

Introduction

Someone you love has been diagnosed as having Alzheimer's disease. If you are like most families, you know very little about this disorder. You don't know what to expect; you don't know what questions to ask; you may not be sure you even want to know. But you have probably heard enough about Alzheimer's disease to be afraid.

Over the last couple of years you may have watched your family member become increasingly dependent, forgetful, and confused. A person whom you have relied upon may now be acting in ways different than you have come to expect. Unpredictable mood changes, such as angry outbursts, may be occurring with increasing frequency, or Mom may show less and less interest in maintaining her typically spotless home. There have been enough changes in the behavior of your family member that you have sought the advice of your physician. You may be concerned that the changes are due to depression, and frequently in the early stages of Alzheimer's disease there is depression as individuals become aware that they are "slipping" and are increasingly forgetful. You may have attributed the changes to other health problems. But now your physician, after a careful examination (see chapter 2), has advised you that the behavior changes are most likely due to Alzheimer's disease. The physician and nursing staff will most likely have discussed with you the nature of this disease, what you can expect, and how it will be treated; they may have even provided you with some written information.

And now you are home. Bits and pieces of your physician's discussion run through your mind. You have a thousand unanswered questions,

9

and you don't know where to start. Until recently little was known regarding Alzheimer's disease and few resources existed to help families with an Alzheimer member. In recent years, more investment in research has occurred: it aims to determine the cause of Alzheimer's disease and to find better ways to manage and treat afflicted patients.

We now have an improved understanding of the deteriorated functioning of the Alzheimer brain. We can only hope that breakthroughs in prevention and treatment are near; but at the present time the assistance that can be provided consists of recommended coping strategies so that: (1) the Alzheimer family member is helped through the progression of this disorder to maintain his/her dignity and as much independence as possible, for as long as possible; and (2) the family caregivers be provided with as much support as possible to remain psychologically and physically healthy, and financially intact. Fortunately there are many agencies in the community and numerous trained professionals to assist family members in their new role as caregivers.

Because Alzheimer's disease affects so many areas of functioning, many disciplines have become involved in conducting research and providing services for victims and their families. This book was developed with the intent of illustrating the many sources of available support. The following chapters combine the collective insights of physicians, nurses, psychologists, social workers, speech pathologists, lawyers, economists, and others who are knowledgeable in the special problems of Alzheimer's disease. The authors have sought to provide practical information for the care of Alzheimer family members, and they have attempted to increase awareness of community resources that may be able to provide even more comprehensive information specifically addressed to each family's unique concerns. This book is designed as an aid in that search for information.

This book was written not only to educate and assist family members of the Alzheimer patient, but to assist the hundreds of thousands of professionals who provide direct care to Alzheimer patients, work with family members of these patients, or provide training or administrative services to those who work with Alzheimer patients. This book is dedicated to all of the heroes, both family members and professional workers, who unselfishly and lovingly provide care for the Alzheimer patient. Few jobs are more emotionally or physically difficult. Caregivers must search inside their hearts for strength and for personal meaning which will enable them to sustain their efforts and to find satisfaction in their humanity.

1

The Caregivers

Raye Lynne Dippel

WHAT IS ALZHEIMER'S DISEASE?

There are over four million people in America who have a dementing illness. According to the Alzheimer's Association, that number is expected to increase to fourteen million within the next fifty years unless a cure or prevention is found. If only five family members are affected for each Alzheimer member, then as many as twenty million Americans may now be facing problems of coping with one of these dreadful diseases. If the physicians, nurses, psychologists, and other professionals who provide care to this special population are added, then the magnitude of the problem and the cost to our society becomes readily apparent.

More than 70 percent of people with Alzheimer's disease live at home. Research suggests that over 75 percent of the home care is provided by family and friends. The additional care necessary generally costs family members $6,000 to $12,000 a year, just to care for the patient at home. Most family members with Alzheimer's disease remain at home until the last and most severe stages of the disease. Nursing home care is very expensive, ranging from $40,000 to $70,000 a year. Neither Medicare nor private health insurance covers the long-term care most patients need. It has been estimated that the average lifetime cost per patient is $174,000. The financial costs of Alzheimer's disease are enormous, but the emotional and physical costs of the disease for the caregiver are of even greater magnitude and are impossible to measure.

Alzheimer's disease is a progressive, degenerative brain disease, which means that with each day that passes the inflicted person becomes more impaired. This degenerative process will eventually result in death, but usually not until the individual has lost his memory, his use of language, his ability to dress or feed himself, and his personality. From the time of diagnosis, the lifespan may range anywhere from three to twenty years. The average is eight years. Men and women are equally affected. Most people affected with Alzheimer's disease are older than age sixty-five. Thus the spouse, who is most frequently the primary caregiver, is often of an age that his or her own health and physical strength may be waning. The caregivers of Alzheimer patients will have ever-increasing demands on their time and their emotional strength. Eventually, individuals with Alzheimer's disease will need twenty-four-hour care. They will need to be dressed, fed, and assisted with toileting. The patient will not recognize his caregiver and may not be able to communicate at even the most basic levels. The patient may wander and get lost. Night and day frequently become confused, with the patient wandering around the house throughout the night, significantly interfering with the sleep of the caregiver. Disturbances in behavior and mood are certain to occur. The Alzheimer patient may become paranoid and aggressive, exploding in angry outbursts, perhaps accusing the caregiver of stealing his shoes or other items that he can no longer find. Clearly things will be much different in this new type of family.

CHANGES IN FUNCTIONAL BEHAVIOR

The Functional Rating Scale for Symptoms of Dementia: This scale was developed by J. Thomas Hutton and his associates to measure changes in everyday behavior, such as eating and dressing, that appeared to be most noticeably affected by the disease. The scale is included here to describe various behaviors that can be expected to change as the disease progresses (see table 1). For example, in the early stages of the disease, the patient may have no difficulty eating with the appropriate utensils. Later, eating with utensils is accomplished with great difficulty, and eventually the patient will need to be fed.

Rate of progression of disease: Scores on the Functional Scale may range from zero (no impairment) to 42 (severe impairment). In a small but interesting study conducted by Dr. Hutton and his colleagues, fourteen Alzheimer patients were monitored over two years. Functional Scale scores were measured every six months throughout the two-year period. At the beginning of the study some patients had only mild impairment (Functional Scale scores of less than 21), while in others, the disease was in its more advanced stages (Functional Scale scores of greater than 21). This study found that Alzheimer's disease caused significantly more impairment in functional ability at each time of measurement. Thus the disease progresses at a relatively stable rate. It would be uncommon, for example, for someone to go for over six months without showing some obvious decline in ability to respond to his environment.

Nursing home placement: During this study, twelve of the fourteen patients were placed in nursing homes by their families. It was discovered that at the time the families decided that they were unable to care for their Alzheimer family member at home, the patient had scores on the Functional Scale in the low 30s. In this study, individuals who had moderate impairment at the beginning of the study were typically placed in nursing homes approximately eighteen to twenty-four months later. Individuals who were more severely impaired at the beginning of the study were typically placed in nursing homes within six months to one year.

There is much variability in the rate of progression of the disease for individual patients. Although life expectancy following the onset of Alzheimer's disease is generally five to ten years, this time may vary widely. The estimates provided here should serve only to aid in planning for eventual nursing home placement. There are sometimes waiting lists for preferred nursing homes, and financial planning will be necessary. Having an idea of when other families have found it necessary to establish residence in a nursing home may help the caregiver to plan for the best possible care for the Alzheimer patient at later stages of the disease. (See chapter 14 for a more in-depth discussion of nursing home placement.)

Several key items on the Functional Scale, (1) incontinence, (2) inability to speak coherently, and (3) the need for assistance with bathing and grooming, were closely associated with institutional placement. By the time an Alzheimer individual is unable to speak coherently, recognize his family, or tend to his own care, the disease has progressed sufficiently that constant supervision and care is required. Other health problems are likely to emerge, increasing the need for skilled nursing care. Once the Alzheimer patient is no longer able to communicate or recognize family members, it may also become easier for the family to *let go* and consider hospitalization as a more emotionally acceptable alternative. There is generally no *one* reason that institutionalization becomes necessary. It is

TABLE 1. FUNCTIONAL RATING SCALE FOR SYMPTOMS OF DEMENTIA

Instructions

1. The scale must be administered to the most knowledgeable informant available. This usually is a spouse or close relative.
2. The scale should be read to the informant one category at a time. The informant is presented the description for behavior in each category. The informant is read each of the responses beginning with zero response. All responses should be read before the informant endorses the highest number response which best describes the behavior of the patient.
3. Responses obtained for each category are summed to give an overall score for functional rating of symptoms of dementia.

Circle the highest number in each category that best describes behavior during the last three months.

Eating:

    0 Eats neatly using appropriate utensils
    1 Eats messily, has some difficulty with utensils
    2 Able to eat solid foods (e.g., fruits, crackers, cookies) with hands only
    3 Has to be fed

Dressing:

    0 Able to dress appropriately without help
    1 Able to dress self with occasional mismatched socks, disarranged buttons or laces
    2 Dresses out of sequence, forgets items, or wears sleeping garments with street clothes—needs supervision
    3 Unable to dress alone, appears undressed in inappropriate situations

Continence:

    0 Complete sphincter control
    1 Occasional bed wetting
    2 Frequent bed wetting or daytime urinary incontinence
    3 Incontinent of both bladder and bowel

Verbal Communication:

    0 Speaks normally
    1 Minor difficulties with speech or word-finding difficulties
    2 Able to carry out only simple, uncomplicated conversations
    3 Unable to speak coherently

Memory for Names:

    0 Usually remembers names of meaningful acquaintances
    1 Cannot recall names of acquaintances or distant relatives
    2 Cannot recall names of close friends or relatives
    3 Cannot recall name of spouse or other living partner

Memory for Events:

    0 Can recall details and sequences of recent experiences
    1 Cannot recall details or sequences of recent events
    2 Cannot recall entire events (e.g., recent outings, visits of relatives or friends) without prompting
    3 Cannot recall entire events even with prompting

Mental Alertness:

  0 Usually alert, attentive to environment
  1 Easily distracted, mind wanders
  2 Frequently asks the same questions over and over
  3 Cannot maintain attention while watching television

Global Confusion:

  0 Appropriately responsive to environment
  1 Nocturnal confusion or confusion upon awakening
  2 Periodic confusion during daytime
  3 Nearly always quite confused

Spatial Orientation:

  0 Oriented, able to find his/her bearings
  1 Spatial confusion when driving or riding in local community
  2 Gets lost when walking in neighborhood
  3 Gets lost in own home or in hospital ward

Facial Recognition:

  0 Can recognize faces of recent acquaintances
  1 Cannot recognize faces of recent acquaintances
  2 Cannot recognize faces of relatives or close friends
  3 Cannot recognize spouse or constant living companion

Hygiene and Grooming:

  0 Generally neat and clean
  1 Ignores grooming (e.g., does not brush teeth and hair, shave)
  2 Does not bathe regularly
  3 Has to be bathed and groomed

Emotionality:

  0 Unchanged from normal
  1 Mild change in emotional responsiveness—slightly more irritable or more passive, diminished sense of humor, mild depression
  2 Moderate change in emotional responsiveness—growing apathy, increased rigidity, despondent, angry outbursts, cries easily
  3 Impaired emotional control—unstable, rapid cycling or laughing in inappropriate situations, violent outbursts

Social Responsiveness:

  0 Unchanged from previous, "normal"
  1 Tendency to dwell on the past, lack of proper association for present situation
  2 Lack of regard for feelings of others, quarrelsome, irritable
  3 Inappropriate sexual acting out or antisocial behavior

Sleep Patterns:

  0 Unchanged from previous, "normal"
  1 Sleeps, noticeably more or less than ,normal
  2 Restless, nightmares, disturbed sleep, increased wakefulness
  3 Up wandering for all or most of the night, inability to sleep

more typically the result of a combination of factors that lead to the primary caregiver becoming *overwhelmed* by the responsibilities.

The Functional Scale may be useful in gathering information regarding the patient's level of functioning, but this information should be combined with all other relevant medical, psychological, social, and economic data before decisions regarding nursing home placement are made. The decision to place a loved one in an institutional setting is perhaps the most difficult decision a family must ever make. Despite the myth that older people are placed in institutions because the family does not care or does not want to be bothered, the opposite is more likely true. It is far more common that an Alzheimer victim is cared for in the home long after the caregiver has exhausted emotional and physical resources.

In between the early stages and the last stages of the disease there will be wide variability in the patient's abilities. Good patient care and management can greatly ease the transitions that the patient and his family will go through. The progression of the disease cannot be modified medically and there is no cure. Education will be the most important means to provide the best quality of life for both the patient and his family. It will assist in making difficult decisions, in finding support from the community, in learning how to structure the home environment to reduce stress and improve patient functioning, in learning how to manage difficult behavior, and perhaps most significantly, learning the importance of taking care of the caregiver.

WHO ARE THE CAREGIVERS?

Caregivers are frequently divided into two categories—*primary* and *secondary*. A primary caregiver is typically the spouse who lives with the demented person. Although estimates vary, one survey reported that 55 percent of caregivers are spouses, 35 percent are adult offspring, 5 percent are siblings, and the remainder are other relatives or paid providers of care. In this study, caregivers ranged in age from the late twenties to the early eighties, with the average age between fifty and seventy. Due to the older age of many of the spouses, caregivers frequently face personal health problems and physical limitations that may increase the difficulty of caring for a demented individual who needs close supervision and assistance in most aspects of daily living.

Following spouses, daughters of Alzheimer victims are the next most likely family members to assume the role of providing primary care. It should be noted that children of Alzheimer patients are typically of an age (thirty to fifty years) at which time they may have additional *roles*, such as childrearing, working outside the home, and other social and community responsibilities. These commitments to spouse and children are important; outside support may therefore be necessary to insure that the family retains the emotional resources needed for optimal growth and development.

Secondary caregivers, who are frequently other relatives, vary greatly in the amount of support and care that they are able to give. Not to be forgotten are the nurses and nurse's aides who provide care for Alzheimer patients on a daily basis, either at home, at a day-care facility, or a nursing home or hospital. Staff burnout and turnover are major problems at institutions that care for Alzheimer patients. Stress, anxiety, and depression are common in these caregivers and cannot be ignored.

STRESS AND THE CAREGIVER

The research on caregivers, which has only recently emerged, is very clear that caregiving is a chronic and persistent stressor, which frequently results in depression, anxiety, and decreased health and well being for the primary caregiver. Secondary caregivers may also suffer significantly. One very interesting study measured the health and well being of almost one hundred spouse primary caregivers, their offspring who were secondary caregivers and who lived near their parents, and the spouses of their offspring, who were also secondary caregivers. The investigators, Lieberman and Fisher, evaluated health and well being in relation to the level of severity of the patient's dementia. Eighty percent of the offspring and in-laws provided care weekly. Daughters provided an average of seven hours of care per week, while sons provided an average of four and a half hours of care per week. Daughters-in-law provided an average of five hours of care per week, and sons-in-law reported caring an average of three hours per week. All three groups of family caregivers showed significant levels of anxiety and depression. Female caregivers reported more anxiety and depression than did male caregivers. Research studies have repeatedly found that female caregivers have a greater vulnerability to depression and anxiety than do their male counterparts. In the general population, females are also more prone to depression and anxiety. Thus, it is not surprising that the additional stressors of providing long-term care would be most distressing to female caregivers, who in general provide more hours of care with less outside help than male caregivers. For example, an elderly man whose wife has Alzheimer's disease may seek more assistance with cooking, shopping, and house care than an elderly woman whose husband has Alzheimer's disease.

In the Lieberman and Fisher study, the spouse caregivers of the Alzheimer patients who had greater levels of behavior impairment experienced more anxiety and depression, more *somatic*, or physical, symptoms, and poorer sense of well being than spouses whose family member was at earlier stages of impairment. Thus, the greater the severity of behavior problems and impairment in daily functioning, the greater the caregiver stress, and the greater the levels of physical symptoms, anxiety, and depression. The adult sons and daughters reported significantly more somatic complaints as their parent's illness became more severe. The more care hours provided, the greater the amount of physical complaints reported. In-law secondary caregivers reported comparable levels of somatic complaints as the offspring which increased as severity of the disease increased. This study demonstrates that all family members suffer from the effects of this disease, that female caregivers are at greatest risk, and that as the number of hours of caregiving increase, caregiver emotional and physical functioning are at risk of becoming impaired.

DEPRESSION AND ANXIETY

Other interesting studies have consistently found that long-term caregivers are at risk of high levels of psychological distress, leading in some cases to psychiatric disorders such as major depression disorder and generalized anxiety disorder, which generally require treatment. Major depression is more than just feeling sad or blue for a few days. It is a serious condition that leaves the individual feeling a loss of pleasure in all activities and pastimes which persists relentlessly over time. The depressed individual may have a poor appetite or significant weight loss, which may complicate health issues in the elderly. There may be disturbances in sleep, loss of energy, fatigue, feelings of worthlessness and guilt, diminished ability to think or concentrate, and sometimes recurrent thoughts of death or suicidal ideation.

Depression may not be readily apparent in the older caregiver. Elderly depressed individuals may not describe themselves as being depressed, preferring instead to suffer silently. They may not be inclined to speak of feelings of despair, poor self-esteem, and worthlessness, and may be less inclined to complain of guilt. Instead, the elderly caregiver may be more likely to complain about feeling tired, loss of energy, sleeplessness, poor appetite, or a vague array of physical problems. The depressed elderly are less prone to tears and may be more likely to express their depression by appearing irritable. It is important to diagnose and treat depression. It can be a fatal disorder, and it is a tragedy for the caregiver to suffer when treatment can greatly relieve the distress and discomfort of depression.

Research studies have reported rates of depression which vary from 10 to 50 percent of the caregivers studied. One study at the University of Washington found that spouse caregivers who have a prior history of psychiatric disorders such as major depression or generalized anxiety disorder were significantly more likely to develop a major depression or other psychiatric disorder while caring for their Alzheimer spouse than did caregivers without a prior history of a psychiatric disorder. Also interesting were findings that the caregivers who had a prior history of depression or anxiety were twice as likely to suffer recurrences than members of the control group who were not Alzheimer caregivers, but who did have a prior history of depression or anxiety.

It will be important to assess carefully and realistically the capacity of the caregiver to provide care. This will need to occur at several points throughout the course of the illness. The person providing care may be successful at managing the patient early in the illness, but as demands increase and the primary caregiver attempts to do more and more, reevaluation of the caregiver's health and resources becomes very important, otherwise it may well be necessary to provide medical care to the caregiver as well. This is especially true for caregivers who have a history of depression and anxiety. Fortunately, depression is a disorder which can be treated with good results. By ensuring that the caregiver has sufficient support, someone to confide in, and plenty of time off, depression may be prevented. If depression is caught and treated early, the caregiver will have much greater physical and emotional strength to cope with the demands of this disorder and may delay the need for nursing home care.

FAMILY STRESSORS

A shift in responsibilities and roles within the family is often necessary when one member assumes the new role of *demented patient*. It may be extremely difficult for the family to divide responsibilities so that the burden does not fall too heavily on the shoulders of any one caregiver. In some cases family conflicts arise, adding anxiety to an already stressful situation. Although little is known about the amount of family conflict and discord associated with Alzheimer's disease, it is likely to be common. Families will vary in their ability to solve problems; some may require outside counselors to assist them (see chapter 6).

Insight into Alzheimer family conflict has been provided by Dr. Jean Scott and colleagues at the Texas Tech Alzheimer's Center. The most frequent family conflicts reported by the primary caregivers include: infrequency of visits from other family members, family members doubting the severity or extent of the illness, and differences in expectations about care. Conflicts over nursing home placement are also reported. Secondary caregivers, on the other hand, reported more conflicts regarding disagreements about treatment of the patient by other family members and the feeling that responsibilities are distributed unfairly among family members.

Interestingly, another study found that some siblings were *excused* from caregiving responsibilities based on their childhood reputations, despite the fact that many had grown into responsible professionals. For example, if the sibling had been identified as *spoiled* or *irresponsible*, or a *problem child*, then family members would not expect the adult sibling to assume caregiving responsibility. Unfortunately these *unencumbered* siblings described a great sense of loss of identity and selfhood. These individuals had more difficulty coming to terms with the loss of their Alzheimer-diseased parent. Family counseling which explores early family history as it relates to current family practices may aid families in distributing the responsibilities of care such that all family members participate not only in the caregiving responsibilities but also in the resolution of feelings of guilt, loss, and grief.

It is important to emphasize that, on the whole, conflicts are not reported in large numbers, but when they are reported they tend to be recurrent and stressful. Frequently the family members do not confront one another about the problems. Most families use open discussion to resolve conflict, but others use avoidance or withdrawal and thus conflicts remain unresolved. As might be expected, the burden of being a caregiver is significantly lighter when no family conflict is present.

COPING STRATEGIES

Stages of Adaptation

Adaptation is a continual process. An individual may go through several stages before successful adaptation is achieved. In the early stages of learning how to cope with a chronic disease, it is common for a person to use denial as a means of controlling fears and anxieties. Denial might take the form of not accepting the diagnosis and avoiding any discussion on the eventual mental decline of a loved one. The patient may be taken to many physicians in an attempt to find another diagnosis or a *cure*. Unproven alternative therapies, such as *vitamin therapy*, may be tried. This stage is usually temporary. As attempts at self-care deteriorate, it becomes progressively more difficult to believe that the patient is *just distracted* or *just depressed*, or that a miracle cure is available.

As the caregiver becomes more accepting of the diagnosis, effort is made to learn as much as possible about the disease. The caregiver begins to develop an awareness of how Alzheimer's disease will change not only the patient's life, but his or her own as well. Feelings of anger emerge regarding the *unfairness* of the disease. Anger is a perfectly normal response to losing control of one's life and destiny. There are few negative events occurring in life that one cannot *change* by working harder or trying something different. The progression of Alzheimer's disease will continue despite efforts on the part of the caregiver. That loss of control will almost invariably intensify feelings of anger, which are particularly difficult to manage, because it is unclear who or what should be the emotional target: the afflicted family member, the health care professional who is turned to for help, or other perplexed family members. Such displaced anger is very likely to result in feelings of guilt. To carry both the anger and the guilt inside without adequate means of expressing these feelings can be highly destructive. It is important to acknowledge the anger and to find someone with whom these feelings can be discussed—a person who will not encourage feelings of guilt.

As time goes by, the anger may continue. The relationship, as the caregiver knew it, with a spouse or a parent has been lost. Life is anything but normal, and intrusive responsibilities pose a heavy burden. However, some measure of control over this life event will have been regained. Armed with information and outside sources of support, family willingness to share the responsibilities, and a better idea of the problems to be faced, the caregiver will possess the tools to manage. This period of reorganization will aid in developing a more *normal* pattern of living. The caregiver will feel more in control, more accepting of this change in his or her life.

With renewed stability and a recognition that the caregiver *will* be able to cope with and manage these challenges, a new stage of adaptation, *resolution,* emerges. During this period, a caregiver may be more successful in reflecting on how his or her life has changed. At this time, those who care for Alzheimer patients may be better able to express emotions, especially sadness and grief. Caregivers are likely to seek out others who have had similar experiences. They may resolve to take better care of their own needs. Caregivers are likely to become more independent, in the sense that more recreational and social activities are sought. Some find other sources of emotional support, such as reaching out to friends or making new ones.

Although actual responsibilities may be increasing and the Alzheimer patient continues to show decline, with successful adaptation the caregiver may actually be more serene than at earlier points in the progression of the disease. Now may be the time to reflect fondly on memories of one's past relationship with the patient and to begin to reconstruct an image of the spouse or parent before the illness took hold. This reconstructed image may actually give comfort and make caregiving a more meaningful and less exasperating experience.

Need for Emotional Support and Time Off

Caregivers report that one of their greatest needs is for emotional support, second only to the need for time off. Many have no one to talk to about the problems they face in caring for a demented family member. The guilt, loss, and grief are especially difficult to express. Caregivers frequently feel that others do not truly understand the extent of care required. Visits from other family members greatly ease the sense of burden. Family members and friends are by far the most common sources of emotional support, although support groups and professionals may assist in relieving feelings of isolation.

Perhaps the most important and valuable coping strategy is the arrangement of an adequate amount of *time off* to run errands and to engage in recreational and social activities. The research is quite clear that individuals who do not obtain a sufficient amount of time away from the responsibilities of caregiving feel a much greater sense of burden and have less success managing their emotional and physical health. Respite care and day care are valuable in this regard. Although community respite and day care have been difficult to find in the past, many cities now have excellent day care programs specifically designed to meet the special needs of Alzheimer patients. If your community does not offer such services, perhaps your local Alzheimer support group can help to develop special day programs (see chapter 12).

Asking for Help

Alzheimer caregivers should learn to be assertive in asking friends and relatives for what they need. Often others would like to help but don't know how. Make a wish list of errands or weekly jobs that need to be done, such as grocery shopping, laundry, dusting, vacuuming, yard work, paying bills, and the like. Other list items might include time spent with the Alzheimer person, such as taking him for a walk or inviting him to help in the garden raking leaves or digging in the dirt. You might ask for supervision of the individual while you attend an Alzheimer support group or go to the movies. Have your list handy and when someone asks how they can help, show them the list and let them help! Many people are too proud to either ask for or accept help. This attitude will make it very difficult for you to sustain the day in and day out care that the Alzheimer individual will require and will deny others the satisfaction of knowing that they have contributed in a significant and meaningful way to the care of the patient and to caring for you as well.

Friends should remember that caregivers may be very busy and tired and may neglect initiating contact with their friends. This does not mean that they do not care about their friendships. Continue to make those phone calls, make those visits, and give those invitations, even if they are not reciprocated. They mean a lot and there will be a time in the future that will allow for greater reciprocity. There is a very large risk for social isolation of the caregiver. If caregivers and their support systems do not actively fight such isolation, the result will be stress, depression, and ill health.

Support Groups

One of the most helpful and important sources of information and emotional support for the caregiver is a local Alzheimer Association support group. Although it may be difficult to attend that first meeting, every person I have ever talked to has told me how important the Alzheimer support group has been in providing information, friendship, and support from others who are going through similar feelings and problems. I strongly suggest that you seek out such an organization as early as possible. (Chapter 12 discusses support groups in more detail.)

Community Resources

Make use of the professionals in your community. They are there to help. Psychologists may assist you in resolving family conflict, reducing behavior problems, making difficult decisions about nursing home placement, and diagnosing and treating depression or anxiety of the caregiver. Physicians and nurses may provide answers regarding medical treatment, nutrition, and safety. Attorneys may be consulted regarding estate planning, guardianship, and living wills. Your local Area Agency on Aging will assist you in obtaining government services. Geriatric care managers, who are usually registered nurses or trained social workers, can assess the needs of elderly people, find services for them, and visit them in their homes. (For help in finding a care manager you can call the National Association of Professional Geriatric Care Managers in Tucson, Arizona, at [520] 881–8008.) Your Alzheimer Association can teach you how to advocate for research and more government assistance for long-term care. Your congressmen and representatives can join you in seeking laws that protect families with catastrophic illnesses.

Not all caregivers seek out the resources that are available in the community. This may be especially true of minority groups, although the incidence of dementia is similar across cultures. In one survey, only 19 percent of minority caregivers had contacted an agency for assistance in locating and arranging services for family members with dementia. Educational materials sensitive to cultural differences and better reach out programs to minorities are needed.

GATHERING INFORMATION

Alzheimer Disease Literature

Besides the useful information you will acquire from your support group, the library and local bookstore will be important places to visit. When this book was first written, there was very little information available to the Alzheimer caregiver. Fortunately, there are now many books and articles addressing this illness. Each one may provide a little more information to assist you in making decisions and managing your life and the life of the patient.

Information from the Internet

An exciting new source of information for Alzheimer caregivers is available from their own homes via their home computer. This is especially helpful to Alzheimer caregivers because getting out of the home can be difficult. With a little help getting started, the caregiver can access the Internet, which is the world's largest computer network. The Internet is aimed at the ordinary computer user, not the expert. There are some small monthly charges to get connected to the Internet via such companies as America Online, Prodigy, Pipeline USA, and others. Once you are *online* you will find many sources of free information on Alzheimer's disease. You will want to access the World Wide Web (WWW or Web) which is an easy link to all the information on the Internet. Your online company will provide you with a Web browser such as Mosaic or Netscape to enter the Web. With your browser you will connect to free search services or companies, such as Lycos, Yahoo, or Excite, through which you will be able to search the entire Internet system for information on Alzheimer's disease. The information is very diverse and may include publications from the Alzheimer's Disease Association, advertisements for books or films, emotional support resources, health news, and many other pieces of information which are far too numerous to cover here.

Through the Web browser or other news reader programs you may also connect with experts or other caregivers on Internet *news groups*. A news group is a group of people who share a common interest, such as Alzheimer's disease. Such a group would share information or communicate with each other by posting news information, asking advice within the group, or by providing their own special knowledge, experience, or information. Through Internet *E-mail* you may ask questions of an individual. For example, through the news group you may find an expert who has done research in an area you are interested in and you may wish to communicate directly and privately with him by E-mail.

Once you have selected your online service and have it installed, using the Internet is really not very complicated and may prove itself to be invaluable to you. Shop around for the best service for you. Some companies charge a monthly fee such as $10 a month then and charge additional fees for any time used after a set number of hours. For example, the company may charge you additional fees for time spent on the Internet over four hours. Other companies may offer unlimited access for a set fee. For example, for $20 a month you may have unlimited access.

CONCLUSION

The individuals that provide for the health, the safety, and the dignity of individuals inflicted with Alzheimer's disease are true heroes. The self-sacrifice that is demanded for extended months is phenomenal. What is most surprising is the willingness, the lack of complaining, and the compassion that thousands and thousands of caregivers demonstrate day after day after day. All caregivers become frustrated. Most provide better care some days than others. Most lose their patience regularly. Most feel angry and resentful at least part of the time. But almost all work desperately to ensure that their loved one ends his days on this earth being loved, nurtured, and cared for in the best possible way. Few caregivers end this process feeling guilt. It is unlikely that caregivers will receive the thanks they deserve, the roses, or the medals. However, the legacy that these individuals leave to their children and grandchildren is the best humanity has to offer and will ensure that future generations will learn about true giving and true love.

SUGGESTED READINGS

Elias, J. E., Hutton, J. T., Bratt, A. H., Miller, B. A., and Weinstein, L. A. "Caretaker Coping and Alzheimer's Patient Decline." *Texas Medicine* 83 (1987): 46–47.

Globerman, J. "The Unencumbered Child: Family Reputations and Responsibilities in the Care of Relatives with Alzheimer's Disease." *Family Process* 34 (1995): 87–99.

Hutton, J. T., Dippel, R. L., Loewenson, R. B., Mortimer, J. A., and Christians, B. L. "Predictors of Nursing Home Placement of Patients with Alzheimer's Disease." *Texas Medicine* 81 (1985): 40–43.

Lieberman, M. A., and Fisher, L. "The Impact of Chronic Illness on the Health and Well-Being of Family Members." *Gerontologist* 35 (1995): 94–102.

O'Quin, J. A., and McGraw, K. O. "The Burdened Caregiver: An Overview." In *Senile Dementia of the Alzheimer's Type,* edited by J. T. Hutton and A. D. Kenny. New York: Alan R. Liss Inc., 1985.

Russo, J., Vitaliano, P. P., Brewer, D. D., Katon, W., and Becker, J. "Psychiatric Disorders in Spouse Caregivers of Care Recipients with Alzheimer's Disease and Matched Controls." *Journal of Abnormal Psychology* 104 (1995): 197–204.

Schulz, R., Visintainer, P., and Williamson, G. M. "Psychiatric and Physical Morbidity Effects of Caregiving." *Journal of Gerontology: Psychological Sciences*, 45 (1990): 181–91.

Scott, J. P., Roberto, K. A., Hutton, J. T., and Slack, D. M. "Family Conflicts in Caring for the Alzheimer's Patient." In *Senile Dementia of the Alzheimer's Type,* edited by J. T. Hutton and A. D. Kenny. New York: Alan R. Liss Inc., 1985.

2

Medical Aspects of Dementia (Senility)

J. Thomas Hutton and Jerry L. Morris

Research on Alzheimer's disease recently has become of utmost importance to our society. Research with Alzheimer patients, however, is not always easy: patients frequently become confused in the new surroundings of a research lab or a doctor's office. It is sometimes difficult to gain compliance with testing during the more advanced stages of the disease. Patients may not understand what is asked of them and may therefore actively resist any effort to get them to "do" something they do not understand.

Despite the difficulties that may arise while testing Alzheimer patients, in the last few years research has greatly expanded our knowledge of this disorder. In what follows, J. Thomas Hutton, a neurologist, and research associate Jerry L. Morris provide an overview of current research findings regarding the brain changes that occur with Alzheimer's disease, the possible causes of this disorder, and the medical interventions that are most beneficial.

The principal form of dementia (senility) is Alzheimer's disease. Whether or not a person is a health care professional, a health care provider, a family member of an Alzheimer victim, or just a taxpayer, there are good reasons for seeking to understand this condition. Alzheimer's disease is very costly. The Alzheimer's Association estimates the cost of the disease in this country to be $80–100 billion each year. This estimate includes the costs of diagnosis, treatment, nursing home care, informal care, and lost income. This staggering financial burden is slated to increase drastically in the next two decades. Approximately four million Americans now have

Alzheimer's disease, and as many as seven million may be afflicted by the year 2010, the year the first of the baby boom generation reaches age sixty-five.

A second important reason for educating ourselves about Alzheimer's disease is that no other chronic medical condition is more devastating to the quality of life. It strips away the personhood of the individual: those human aspects that are held most dear—the ability to think, to plan, to remember, and to function as a productive member of society—are taken away.

A third reason for attributing so much importance to Alzheimer's disease is its status as a major killer, ranking fourth or fifth among our nation's most frequent causes of death. It is known that a person diagnosed as having Alzheimer's disease will, on average, live only one-third to one-half as long as a person of the same age who does not have the disease. If this increased mortality rate is combined with the incidence of the disease in the general population, it can be demonstrated that Alzheimer's disease is a principal cause of death, with only heart disease, cancer, and stroke taking a higher toll of human life. However, it is rare to see Alzheimer's disease listed on a death certificate: more typically, pneumonia is indicated as the cause of death in the Alzheimer victim. It is logical to assume that the fatal infection would not have been contracted were it not for the debilitated state that directly resulted from the Alzheimer's disease.

The prevalence, cost, and suffering that result from Alzheimer's disease will increase dramatically over the next forty years unless the cause and the cure are found. This increase will result from a doubling of the population of older persons within our society. The subgroup that will show the most rapid increase in population is those persons over the age of eighty-five years. These oldest of the old have the highest risk for developing Alzheimer's disease. It is also these oldest of the old who are at risk for contracting other chronic diseases, all of which increase the need for nursing homes. This will place an increased burden on such facilities.

At present, it is estimated that 40 to 60 percent of the nation's nursing home residents suffer from dementia (senility). Of those individuals with dementia, the majority are victims of Alzheimer's disease. Only recently has the significance of this disease entered the public's consciousness. We have begun to realize that with the aging of our society, America will soon be confronted with an epidemic of age-related medical problems, the most devastating of which will be Alzheimer's disease.

DEFINITION OF DEMENTIA

The term *dementia* refers to an across-the-board decline in intellectual abilities. This is an acquired disorder as compared to disorders present at birth, such as mental retardation. Dementia is strongly linked to age, becoming progressively more frequent with advancing age and is assumed to be due to brain impairment.

Dementia is not a diagnosis but a broad symptom complex and can result from a variety of causes. It may or may not be reversible depending upon the underlying cause. The symptoms of dementia consist of disorientation, poor memory, reduced intellectual functioning, reduced judgment, and alterations in emotional background. Implicit in the definition of dementia is loss of everyday skills.

EVALUATION OF DEMENTED PERSONS

Persons who develop symptoms of dementia should undergo a medical evaluation for treatable causes. Even if a treatable form of dementia is not found, it is advantageous to establish a diagnosis because this makes it possible to predict the course of the particular illness.

The evaluation begins with a history of the illness and is usually obtained from a family member or close friend since the demented individual is no longer capable of providing accurate information. For diagnostic purposes the physician will be very interested to know when symptoms began to occur: certain diseases, such as Alzheimer's disease, have a slow and insidious onset. Rarely is it possible for the family member to date precisely the beginning of this dementing illness. In contrast, symptoms may have arisen quite suddenly if the patient has a disorder such as liver failure, kidney failure, or drug overdose.

The course of the dementing illness, or the rate at which symptoms become more severe, is also meaningful. In the case of Alzheimer's disease, the course is invariably slow and progressive. Alzheimer's disease will usually progress for several years prior to becoming severe enough that the family will seek medical attention. The victim may in the early stages have a tacit awareness that something is amiss, although frequently the affected person is without any appreciation of these potential problems. So-called multi-infarct dementia is caused by serial strokes. Unlike Alzheimer's disease, this form of dementia presents a pattern of step-by-

TABLE 1

CAUSES OF DEMENTIA SYNDROME

Alzheimer's disease
Pick's disease
Multi-infarct dementia
Bilateral subdural hematomas (blood clots on the brain)
Brain tumors, especially involving the frontal lobes
Chronic fungal or tuberculous meningitis
Kidney failure
Liver failure
Electrolyte imbalance
Drug overdosage
Hypo- or hyperthyroidism
Hydrocephalous
Huntington's disease
Late Multiple Sclerosis
Late Parkinson's disease
Post-traumatic brain injury
Depression
Chronic alcoholism
Pernicious anemia
Neurosyphilis
Creutzfeldt-Jakob disease
AIDS

step progression punctuated by the occurrence of multiple strokes. In between the strokes victims may actually improve slightly.

The history of fluctuations in alertness is also helpful. The Alzheimer victim will normally have an alert level of consciousness. In contrast, persons suffering from liver failure, kidney failure, drug overdosage, blood clots on the brain (subdural hematomas), electrolyte imbalance, or infections of the nervous system will typically have fluctuating periods of alertness and sleepiness.

In addition to a medical history, both general and neurological examinations should, be performed. Their purpose is to find impairment of organ systems or evidence of localized brain disease. For example, the physician may find evidence of liver or kidney failure (fluctuating level of consciousness, flapping type of tremor of outstretched hands, and unusual odor). The physician may also find evidence of localized disease

---

TABLE 2

LABORATORY TESTS

Blood count
Urinalysis
metabolic screen (SMA–12 or AA-chem)
Thyroid tests
Syphilis screen (RPR or VDRL)
B–12 level
Drug screen for hypnotic agents
CT or MRI scan of head
Electroencephalogram
Cerebrospinal fluid analysis
HIV testing

---

of the brain, as may be seen with a brain tumor or a blood clot. Alternatively, the physician may find evidence of multiple areas of the brain and brainstem that are injured as is typically the case with multi-infarct dementia. Careful general and neurological examinations may suggest various diagnostic possibilities that can then be systematically investigated.

Many different disease processes can give rise to the dementia syndrome. Table 1 provides a partial list of medical entities known to be capable of giving rise to dementia.

Useful Laboratory Tests

Following the history and physical examination, a battery of laboratory tests is performed, the purpose of which is to gain additional diagnostic information. The laboratory tests may have been prompted by the history or the physical examination, or they may simply be conducted to exclude the possibility of a particular disorder. Table 2 lists laboratory tests that may be used to uncover more treatable forms of dementia.

Other laboratory tests such as cerebral angiography, skull X-rays, serum ammonia, scinticisternography (a radioactive agent is injected into the spinal fluid to determine if occult hydrocephalous exists), and nuclear brain scans may be performed.

Outcome of Evaluation for Treatable Forms of Dementia

Large numbers of patients presenting symptoms of dementia have been evaluated to determine the frequency of treatable forms. These studies have found that from 10 to 20 percent of persons with symptoms of dementia have underlying diseases for which specific treatments exist. It is the physician's first responsibility to identify those individuals with potentially reversible forms of dementia. Though the cost of performing a medical screen is not cheap, this examination is substantially less than the cost of a nursing home. In addition, the possibility of finding a disease which, if treated, would return the patient to a more normal mental state fully warrants the cost and the effort.

TREATMENT

If a potentially reversible form of dementia is found, then the treatment logically follows. For example, if a brain tumor is discovered, then surgery, radiation therapy, or chemotherapy would be prescribed. Similarly appropriate therapy would follow for the various endocrine (glandular), metabolic, or toxic disorders.

Whereas only one out of five patients is found to have a specific underlying cause for which treatment is available, the physician is frequently limited to providing therapy to treat the symptoms. Certain symptoms of dementia may respond to medicine or behavioral therapy. Depression frequently accompanies dementia, especially in the early stages. Depression can by itself give rise to a dementia syndrome and may respond favorably if treated. An antidepressant medication is typically prescribed. Various antidepressants act as sedatives while others serve to stimulate. A medication best suited to the patient's needs will be chosen.

Another symptom that may arise, especially in the late phases of dementia, is *sundowning*: a person will become confused late in the day, i.e., when the sun goes down. The individual may become agitated and violent as well. A small dose of a tranquilizer will usually suffice to control the situation if behavioral intervention does not prove successful. The most widely used tranquilizers for dementia are thioridazine (Mellaril), chlorpromazine (Thorazine), haloperidol (Haldol), thiothixine (Navane), and clozapine (Clozaril). All of these agents have potential side effects, one of the most bothersome and potentially dangerous of which is the occurrence

TABLE 3

DRUGS IN DEVELOPMENT FOR ALZHEIMER'S DISEASE (U.S.)

Drug	Company	Status
AF102B	Forest Laboratories	Phase III
ALCAR (acetyl-l-carnitine)	Sigma-Tau Pharmaceuticals	Phase III
BIIP-20	Boehringer Ingelheim	Phase II
DHEA (dihydroepiandrosterone)	Neurocrine Biosciences	Phase II
E2020	Eisai; Pfizer	Phase III
eptastigmine (MF–201)	Mediolanum Pharmaceuticals	Phase II
milameline	Warner-Lambert	Phase III
propentofylline	Hoechst-Roussel Pharmaceuticals	Phase III
Reminyl™ (sabeluzole)	Janssen Pharmaceutical	Phase III
SB202026	SmithKline Beecham	Phase II
SDZ ENA–713	Sandoz Pharmaceuticals	Phase III
Sermion® (nicergoline)	Pharmacia & Upjohn	Phase II
SR 46559	Sanofi	Phase II
SR 57746	Sanofi	Phase II
Synapton (physostigmine)	Forest Laboratories	Phase III
xanomeline (LY 246708)	Eli Lilly	Phase II

Copyright © 1996 Pharmaceutical Research & Manufacturers of America

of a Parkinsonian-like state. The increase in muscle tone, tremor, and poor balance can give rise to functional disability. Of the major tranquilizers, clozapine (Clozaril) has the least tendency to give rise to Parkinsonian symptoms; however, it does pose a significant risk for the development of agranulocytosis, a dangerous drop in the white blood cell count. Careful monitoring of the white cell count is required during treatment with clozapine (Clozaril). Sudden drops in blood pressure with resultant fainting can occur with thioridazine (Mellaril) and chlorpromazine (Thorazine).

It should be emphasized that most behavioral outbursts can be handled without medication. Routine dosages of the major tranquilizers are usually not required and should not be employed in lieu of nurses or therapists.

A variety of medications have been marketed as dilators (expanders) of brain arteries. Such agents are papaverine and cyclandelate. These agents were originally marketed when it was believed that the usual forms of dementia were caused by "hardening of the arteries." It is now known that the principal form of dementia, Alzheimer's disease, has no more arteriosclerosis than would be expected based on age. The vasodilators therefore have a poor rationale and are now used infrequently.

Another category of medication is that of the metabolic enhancers, the best-known agent being a combination of ergoloid mesylates (Hydergine). This agent, while not impressive in its results, does have a substantial body of literature to suggest that it may be of mild benefit for some of the symptoms of dementia. A trial of this agent usually extends over several months to determine whether it may be of benefit. A realistic assessment of the value of such medications focuses on whether or not they slow the expected rate of decline. Some believe that the ergoloid mesylates may favorably alter the rate of disease progression.

Lecithin or choline have been used in the attempt to increase the brain chemical acetylcholine, which is known to be reduced in Alzheimer's disease. Lecithin and choline are building blocks in the formation of acetylcholine. Tacrine hydrochloride (Cognex) acts to reduce the breakdown of acetylcholine. Initial study reports purported to show impressive gains in cognitive performance and everyday activities of daily living with the use of tacrine (Cognex). Unfortunately, results from large-scale clinical trials were not as impressive. Tacrine (Cognex) may be beneficial to some patients with mild to moderate disease; however, the drug does not stop the progression of the disease and any benefit derived can be expected to deteriorate with time. Realistically, the most that should be expected is a slowing in the progress of the disease by a few months in some patients. Tacrine (Cognex) is approved by the U.S. Food and Drug Administration for the treatment of Alzheimer's disease.

Recently, the Pharmaceutical Research and Manufacturers of America listed sixteen drugs in development for Alzheimer's disease (see table 3). Eight of these agents were in phase III clinical trials, that is, tests of the effectiveness of the drug in large numbers of patients with Alzheimer's disease.

BRAIN CHANGES IN ALZHEIMER'S DISEASE

When Alois Alzheimer described in 1907 the disorder that now bears his name, he did so by describing microscopic brain abnormalities. These brain changes consist of neuritic (senile) plaques and neurofibrillary tangles. Neuritic plaques are believed to be degenerating treelike branchings of brain cells that may surround a central core of protein (amyloid). Neurofibrillary tangles are seen within brain cells and consist of a coarsening and thickening of the usually delicate filaments (threadlike tissues). Increasing numbers of neuritic plaques and neurofibrillary tangles correspond to increasing severity of dementia. They may also be seen in normal older brains, but in lesser numbers.

POSSIBLE CAUSES OF ALZHEIMER'S DISEASE

The cause for Alzheimer's disease is unknown. The ultimate solution for the many problems that result from this disorder is to find the cause(s) and to prevent the disease. At present several intriguing possibilities exist. The genetic, unconventional virus, aluminum, and autoimmune hypotheses will be discussed.

The Genetic Hypothesis

Alzheimer's disease is not a strongly genetic disorder such as diabetes mellitus or Huntington's disease, nevertheless a slight genetic risk for Alzheimer's disease results from the presence of a family member with the disease. The risk for the family member of an Alzheimer victim may be strongly influenced by the age of onset of the disease. For example, Alzheimer's disease that has its onset at age forty may present a 40 percent risk for family members. In contrast, Alzheimer's disease beginning after the age of eighty brings about little or no increase for the family member as compared to the general population.

Family members of Alzheimer victims frequently ask whether they are at increased risk for developing the disease. Unfortunately, at present no good predictor exists as to who will develop the disease. In addition, the typical late onset of Alzheimer's disease makes it impossible to carry out effective family planning. At present the best advice that can be offered is a rough estimate of risk based on the age of onset of Alzheimer's disease in the affected family member.

One additional piece of evidence suggesting that Alzheimer's disease may have a genetic basis comes from the study of mentally retarded persons with Down's syndrome. This genetic disorder results from an extra number 21 chromosome (trisomy 21). It is now known that Down's syndrome individuals will develop brain neuritic plaques and neurofibrillary tangles by the age of forty. The strong association between Alzheimer's disease and Down's syndrome, the latter of which is clearly known to be genetic in origin, suggests that a genetic mechanism may also be at work in Alzheimer's disease.

Some early onset familial Alzheimer's disease has been associated with a rare mutation of amyloid precursor protein on chromosome 21. More recently, a mutated gene on chromosome 14 has been linked to early onset Alzheimer's disease. This mutation may account for the majority of the relatively rare early onset familial Alzheimer's disease.

The vast majority of Alzheimer's cases are late-onset (past age sixty-five). Late-onset Alzheimer's disease has recently been linked to a defect on chromosome 19. This defect is in a gene for a blood plasma protein known as apolipoprotein (ApoE) that is involved with cholesterol transport. ApoE is also secreted in the brain and it is associated with the neuritic plaques and neurofibrillary tangles found in the brains of Alzheimer's patients. one variant of the ApoE gene (ApoE4) correlates strongly with late-onset disease, both the familial and sporadic types. Late-onset Alzheimer's disease is most likely caused by multiple factors. There are healthy, elderly people with the ApoE4 gene, and there are Alzheimer victims who do not have the ApoE4 gene. Thus, ApoE4 is probably best described as a susceptibility gene or risk factor for late development of Alzheimer's disease. There is now a test to identify the presence of this gene in DNA taken from a small sample of blood. This test may provide useful information in assessing susceptibility to late-onset Alzheimer's disease.

Three genes on three separate chromosomes (14, 19, and 21) have now been associated with Alzheimer's disease. This represents an important step in identifying the genetic basis for the disease and offers the possibility of medical screening and potentially the treatment of individuals at risk.

The Unconventional Virus Hypothesis

The strongest evidence linking Alzheimer's disease to an unconventional "slow" virus infection results from the discovery that other rare neurological diseases previously thought to be degenerative in nature have now been shown to be caused by transmissible viruslike agents. The rare neurological diseases that now fall into this category consist of Kuru, Scrapie (a disease of sheep), and Creutzfeldt-Jakob disease. Kuru and Creutzfeldt-Jakob disease both cause dementia in humans. Transmission experiments have been carried out which consist of taking a Kuru, Scrapie, or Creutzfeldt-Jakob brain and injecting the filtered tissue into the brains of animals. These experiments have demonstrated, after a latency of many years, that the neurological disease could be transmitted to the animal.

Substantial effort has been expended in an attempt to transmit Alzheimer's disease to nonhuman primates, such as chimpanzees, but without success. Some investigators believe that failure to transmit the disease may result from an unsuitable host; they do not believe that the inability to transmit precludes the possibility that Alzheimer's disease is caused by an unconventional viruslike agent.

What does seem clear is that persons exposed to Alzheimer victims do not have an increased chance of developing the disease. Although special procedures are necessary for handling the blood and cerebrospinal fluid of patients with Creutzfeldt-Jakob disease, no such precautions are deemed necessary for Alzheimer's disease.

The Aluminum Hypothesis

Scientific claims have been made that the brains of Alzheimer victims contain increased amounts of aluminum. Also the feeding of large amounts of aluminum to laboratory animals has been shown to bring about neurofibrillary tangles, which is one of the characteristic microscopic features of Alzheimer's disease. These reports have in the past received substantial coverage in the popular press and have given rise to great concern regarding the usage of aluminum cookware, drinking water in which aluminum was used in the purification process, or even breathing air containing substantial amounts of aluminum.

The aluminum hypothesis has been seriously questioned. The neurofibrillary tangles associated with aluminum, when examined under the electron microscope, appear different from those seen in Alzheimer's disease. In addition, other scientists have not been able to replicate the findings of increased amounts of aluminum in the brains of Alzheimer victims. A general loss of enthusiasm for the aluminum hypothesis has thus occurred in recent years, although the role of aluminum or other environmental agents as a cause or facilitator of the disease does remain a possibility (see chapter 6 for additional information).

The Autoimmune Hypothesis

The immune system declines with advanced age. Despite this overall decline in immune function, increased numbers of antibodies that react to brain proteins develop in older animals and humans. This suggests the possibility that Alzheimer's disease may be caused by the immune system attacking the brain. Other autoimmune diseases, such as rheumatoid arthritis, are known to increase with advancing years as does Alzheimer's disease.

One problem with the autoimmune hypothesis is that the brain is normally protected from the peripheral circulation by a semipermeable barrier referred to as the blood-brain barrier. This barrier may become leaky with age allowing for sensitization or passage of brain-reactive antibodies into the central nervous system. Also, many insults (conditions) exist, such as concussion, chronic hypertension, stroke, or alcoholism, that are known to damage the blood-brain barrier. This suggests the possibility that an environmental insult or disease may be necessary to damage the barrier, giving rise to the possibility of developing Alzheimer's disease. Some recent animal research has shown that brain-reactive antibodies typically layer out in the small arteries of the brain. When a chemical is injected that opens the blood-brain barrier, such antibodies enter the brain and attach especially to the larger brain cells and in brain areas quite reminiscent of Alzheimer's disease. The autoimmune hypothesis, although attractive, is far from proven.

CONCLUSION

A number of exciting developments exist with regard to possible causes of Alzheimer's disease. Only within the last fifteen to twenty years has this disease received any appreciable degree of research interest. New research developments are occurring at an increasing rate. It is hoped that continued research on Alzheimer's disease will lead to effective treatment and prevention of this serious neurological disorder.

SUGGESTED READINGS

Davis, K. L., and Mobs, R. C. "Cholinergic Drugs in Alzheimer's Disease." *New England Journal of Medicine* 315 (1986): 1286–87.

Fraser, V., and Thornton, S. M. *Understanding Senility: A Layperson's Guide.* Amherst, N.Y.: Prometheus Books, 1987.

Hutton, J. T. "Focus Issue: Alzheimer's Disease." *Texas Medicine* 83 (1987): 6–10, 20–64.

Mace, N. L., and Rabins, P. V. *The Thirty-Six Hour Day.* Baltimore: Johns Hopkins University Press, 1981.

Rowe, J. W., and Besdine, R. W. *Health and Disease in Old Age.* Boston: Little, Brown, and Company, 1982.

Saunders, A. M., et al. "Association of Apolipoprotein E Allele E4 with Late-onset Familial and Sporadic Alzheimer's Disease." *Neurology* 43 (1993): 1467–72.

3

Exercise and Aging

Berry N. Squyres

A major task of caregivers is to encourage activity and autonomy in Alzheimer patients. One caregiver was very pleased that her husband continued to enjoy gardening. One day, however, a neighbor's dog dug up the plants he had just put out. As Alzheimer patients will sometimes do when events happen that they cannot understand, this man came to an erroneous conclusion. He decided that his neighbor had dug up his plants. Using the premise that turnabout is fair play, he went next door and removed his neighbor's plants! Gardening continued to be an important source of exercise and activity for this man, and the neighbor forgave him.

In this chapter Dr. Squyres discusses the importance of exercise for both health and emotional well-being. He suggests that exercise is an activity to be enjoyed by the caregiver and the patient together!

It is well known that the population of the United States is rapidly aging. As greater numbers get older, there is an increase in the number of people who develop dementia. By far the most common dementia is Alzheimer's disease (see chapter 2), and there are also the less frequently occurring dementias, such as those associated with small strokes resulting from arteriosclerosis (so-called hardening of the arteries). The treatment of dementia becomes one that must be approached from many perspectives. The patient, the patient's family, the family doctor, other medical specialists, social workers, home health providers, and physiotherapists must work together to improve the general outlook for the patient. The goals of treatment include maintaining the physical health of the patient by treating other diseases that may worsen the dementia, alleviating dementia symptoms whenever possible, and providing a social and physical environment that will allow the highest possible level of functioning.

Although there are few specific studies of exercise programs for individuals with dementia, a number of studies have been conducted that show that a routine exercise program benefits people of all ages, particularly older individuals. Although it is optimal to start an exercise program in the younger years and to continue throughout adulthood, it is never too late to begin exercising.

A sedentary lifestyle presents a definite risk for heart and blood vessel disease. There are many areas of *normal aging* that are really not aging at all but due to inactivity. It has been proven that forced inactivity (illness or incapacity) has many of the same characteristics of so-called *normal aging*. These include increased loss of bone calcium, decrease in oxygen use, decrease in the output (the amount of blood pumped per beat) of the heart, decrease in red blood cells (anemia), and a decrease in glucose tolerance (tendency to diabetes mellitus). Decreased activity is also associated with increased blood pressure, increased body fat, and elevated cholesterol levels.

It is important to note that health benefits can be shown at relatively low levels of activity. The greatest improvement demonstrated is between the least active individuals and those who are moderately active: in other words, from no activity to some activity, however minor. Much less beneficial effect is apparent between the moderately active and the very active.

To reach true fitness for the heart and blood vessels, the aging patient should have fifteen to twenty consecutive minutes of exercise at least three times per week. The exercise should be of an intensity that increases the heart rate to 75 percent of its maximum rate. The maximum heart rate can be calculated roughly by subtracting one's age from 220. The goal is to reach 75 percent of this figure (or 220 − age × .75). There should always be a careful physical evaluation of any individual past the age of forty who undertakes an exercise program. This evaluation is more important as one grows older and even more important for the demented elderly. However, since this level of exercise will be difficult or impossible to attain in the patient with Alzheimer's disease or multi-infarct dementia, a careful physical examination without a stress test would be acceptable if the patient is unable to take such a test.

HEART AND BLOOD VESSEL BENEFITS

It is generally accepted that the most important heart and blood vessel benefit that comes about from regular exercise is increased usage of oxygen, which improves heart muscle efficiency and decreases the likelihood of hypertension (high blood pressure). The best overall way to measure fitness is to measure maximum oxygen uptake, or the amount of oxygen that can be used in a measured period of time. An exercise program helps the use of oxygen by increasing the heart's output, and also by increasing the usage of oxygen by the muscles and other organs. Exercise brings about a decrease in the resting systolic blood pressure (the pressure when the heart beats) and diastolic blood pressure (pressure between beats). This reduction of blood pressure is better when it can come about by what has been called *hygienic means* such as exercise, reduction of weight, decreased salt intake, and psychological behavioral treatment rather than by the use of medication.

MUSCLE, BONE, AND JOINT BENEFITS

At least two significant advantages of exercise accrue to the musculoskeletal system. One is that with increased muscle endurance, muscle fatigue is reduced. Another is the treatment and prevention of osteoporosis. The latter is a decrease in bone mass or density that comes with aging and is particularly prevalent in women after menopause.

Although the reversal of osteoporosis is not to be expected, its progression can be stopped. There are physicians who believe that some rebuilding of bone may occur with proper diet and exercise. Ten percent of women age fifty have suffered broken bones due to osteoporosis. By the age of eighty, 25 percent of all women have sustained hip fractures. Studies both in experimental animals and humans have indicated that physical activity slows or prevents bone loss that occurs in many menopausal women. Osteoporosis is facilitated by decreased activity, decreased hormones, and inadequate diet (low caloric and calcium intake). It has been shown that exercise can be of benefit even without changing diet or hormonal states, although a comprehensive treatment program would address all three areas. It is noteworthy that the average adult needs 1500 mg. of elemental calcium per day (see chapter 6). It is very difficult to obtain this level of calcium in the diet. Therefore, one should consider augmenting one's diet with a calcium supplement. It is vital to understand that we speak of *elemental calcium*. The total weight of the calcium compound is given on the label of medications, but the level of elemental calcium can also be found on the label.

It is important when discussing the bone, joint, and muscle benefits of exercise that emphasis be given to stretching exercises, which are a vital part of every comprehensive exercise program and may be even more important for the demented patient. Stretching exercises ensure increased flexibility of the joints, which may help to prevent injury (i.e., reduces risk of falling). Stretching exercises also improve coordination and efficiency. There is an increase in strength of the tendons, and the bone is stronger because of repetitive use.

METABOLIC BENEFITS

Two major benefits of exercise have been demonstrated in the body's metabolism. One is the increase in high density lipoprotein cholesterol (HDL-C), and the other is increased glucose tolerance, or reduction of the likelihood of diabetes mellitus.

Three major types of cholesterol exist: lipoprotein cholesterol (HDL-C), low-density lipoprotein cholesterol (LDL-C), and very low density lipoprotein cholesterol (VLDL-C). The latter two are harmful and speed up the process of hardening of the arteries. High density lipoprotein cholesterol slows this process and has been demonstrated to offset some of the effects of the other two. Even moderate exercise has been shown to produce significantly higher levels of HDL-C than those values seen with inactive subjects. Walking is quite beneficial in this regard.

Physical exercise improves glucose tolerance and decreases the amount of insulin required (even in those with well-controlled diabetes mellitus). Routine exercise programs aid the prevention and treatment of diabetes mellitus for all patients, including those age sixty-five and older.

PSYCHOLOGICAL BENEFITS

Even after a single exercise session, definite psychological benefits are present. Regular or routine exercise is better still. Research has shown a definite reduction in muscle tension associated with exercise. Also, evidence exists that anxiety or nervousness decreases with exercise. Moderate exercise has been shown to be especially effective in the treatment of depression. Increased thinking capacity may occur with exercise of moderate intensity. This improvement in thinking ability is believed to be above and beyond the help that comes from the lowering of anxiety and tension, and from the decreased depression. The absence of depression is one of the most quickly recognized differences between physically active and sedentary men.

In demented individuals, a regular exercise program may reduce restlessness and agitation and improve mood. Since the patient should always be accompanied by an attendant, an exercise routine followed by the caregiver will be physically and psychologically beneficial to both. Whereas motor skills are preserved to a much greater extent in Alzheimer's disease than are cognitive and memory skills, the demented individual may still be able to perform with some degree of competence and self-satisfaction. It is also an excellent opportunity for the caregiver and patient to interact socially.

SUGGESTED EXERCISE REGIMEN

Ideally, the exercise program should be carried out at least three times a week (daily if possible). The routine should begin with eight to ten minutes of stretching exercises. For some patients this part of the program may be all that is feasible, and this time may be extended to include the entire exercise program. The stretching exercises might include the arms and shoulders, the hips, the knees, and the ankles. Side bends, toe touches, sit-ups, leg lifts, and other familiar exercises are to be encouraged if possible. In the greatly incapacitated patient, the stretching exercises can be performed for the patient by the caregiver in a passive fashion, although this is not as beneficial as are the active exercises.

After the stretching period, whenever possible, a twelve- to thirty-minute aerobic exercise program should begin. This may include walking, stationary cycling, or other exercises of this type. In inclement weather, walking may be done inside the house or, in this present day and age, at the nearest mall, where the temperature is usually in a satisfactory range. Milder forms of exercise may be all that can be done. These might include extending and rotating the arms or holding on to a chair and alternately swinging one leg and then the other.

The exercise program, if it is strenuous enough to produce an increased heart rate, an increased breathing rate, and significant perspiration or sweating, should be followed by a cooldown period of at least four to six minutes. The patient should be kept moving during this time. The stretching exercises mentioned earlier are very important at this time also.

CONCLUSION

It is believed that one way to achieve maximum function for the patient with Alzheimer's disease and multi-infarct dementia is an individualized exercise program. The active involvement and participation of the caregiver in the program is recommended and will provide positive health benefits for both.

SUGGESTED READINGS

Emes, C. "The Effects of a Regular Program of Light Exercise in Seniors." *Journal of Sports Medicine and Physical Fitness* 19 (1979): 195–98.

Engel, G. "The Clinical Applications of the Biopsychosocial Model." In *Elderly Patients and Their Doctors,* edited by M. Haug. New York: Springer Publishing, 1981.

Gluck, F. "Exercises in the Elderly—Benefits, Precautions and Recommendations." *Journal of Tennessee Medical Association* 78 (1985): 162–63.

Lonnerblod, L. "Exercises to Promote Independent Living in Older Patients." *Geriatrics* 39 (1984): 93–101.

Yeater, R., and Martin, R. "Senile Osteoporosis: The Effects of Exercise." *Postgraduate Medicine* 75 (1984): 147–59.

4

Optimal Living Environments for Alzheimer Patients

Jo Ann L. Shroyer and J. Thomas Hutton

An Alzheimer patient may have lived in his home for over thirty years but still be unable to find his way from the living room to the bathroom. Imagine having memory problems and then moving to a nursing home where all the doors and rooms along the hall look the same. How would you ever find your way to the restroom in time?

One woman who had a very close relationship with her husband (who was in the early stages of Alzheimer's disease) recalls accompanying her husband to her sister's house. He had gone to the restroom and had been gone for some time. She finally heard his voice calling from the other side of the house, "Honey, I'm lost. Come find me." The wife reports having been touched by his faith in her to take care of him at that particular time and throughout his illness.

Part of caring for the Alzheimer patient is to reduce the level of stress as much as possible by providing an environment that the patient can successfully negotiate and one in which he feels secure. Dr. Jo Ann L. Shroyer and Dr. J. Thomas Hutton provide ideas on how to modify the home environment or the nursing home environment to better meet the needs of an individual with Alzheimer's disease.

INTRODUCTION

Several programs have been instituted since the 1950s to provide better housing and facilities for the elderly. However, many housing facilities

47

have been designed and constructed with little knowledge of the biological characteristics of aging persons. Additionally, most policies and standards relative to the design of buildings by architects, environmental planners, interior designers, and others have been formulated on the basis of assumption, rather than information obtained through systematic research that includes user needs. As a result, living environments frequently are not responsive to the needs of older people, particularly persons suffering from dementia of the Alzheimer type. Several environmental variables, including illumination, noise abatement, color, furnishings, spatial arrangement, pattern, and texture are consistently deficient. Any one of these features, if problematic or inappropriately applied, can further complicate the life of an individual experiencing dementia. Certain environmental design features may not only threaten the person's health, safety, and welfare, but produce anxiety that can amplify cognitive deficits and result in negative behavioral responses.

PHYSICAL AND COGNITIVE DEFICITS

Human beings are well known for their adaptability to various living environments; however, the design of a living environment has important consequences for individuals with Alzheimer's disease. Indeed, the effectiveness of living environments in making life tasks manageable is directly related to both an individual's mental and physical ability. Therefore, ability, as related to the negotiation of the environment, may be increasingly difficult for Alzheimer patients to achieve as a result of changes in brain function.

Although the role of the environment in the treatment of Alzheimer patients has been explored, evidence suggests that impaired orientation, visual disturbances, impaired memory, and physical impairment can be compensated for somewhat by the design and grouping of environmental stimuli.

Orientation Impairment

Alzheimer patients who are experiencing impaired orientation with regard to time and place normally lack critical judgment (interpreting physical environments is an abstract function), have varying degrees of memory dysfunction, are confused, have personality changes, and have a loss of language skills. Caregivers and designers should consider several design elements when planning environments to help compensate for these deficits. The elements to be considered include illumination, color, furnishings, and signage.

Illumination

• Increase the intensity of lighting during daylight hours and decrease the intensity during evening and night hours to reduce confusion relative to time.

• Provide low light (e.g., a small night-light) in bedrooms, bathrooms, and hallways during night hours to provide information relative to place.

Color

• Color may be used to assist the individual in identifying important places: in nursing homes where many corridors look the same and the halls have similar doors, finding a restroom, or even a resident's own room, can be particularly difficult. Painting all restroom doors a contrasting color to walls and bedroom doors, for example, may aid the person in accessing the facility and thereby reduce the incidence of incontinence.

Furnishings

• Furnishing should clearly denote the nature of activities to reduce confusion and promote individual autonomy (e.g., dining rooms should not also be used for activity areas).

• Use sound-absorbent materials in all areas; emphasize use of sound-retardant materials in corridors and dining areas to reduce audio confusion.

• Although clutter is to be avoided, both at home and in nursing homes, familiar objects (e.g., family pictures, a favorite chair, a familiar bedspread) should be used to assist with orientation.

Signs

- The use of appropriately placed and labeled signs can improve orientation. Signs should be prepared with large letters and placed at eye level on the walls. When possible, graphic illustrations should be used (e.g., female figure or male figure on restroom door).
- Large clocks and calendars prominently displayed can facilitate time orientation.

Visual Disturbance

Individuals who have been diagnosed as having Alzheimer's disease may also experience visual problems. Visual disturbances include decreased depth perception, increased sensitivity to glare, reduced sensitivity to glare, reduced sensitivity for distinguishing subtle contrast, blurred vision, and shrinkage of the visual field. To compensate for these deficits, design elements should include appropriate illumination, contrasting color palette, color, uncluttered spatial furniture arrangement, and simplistic patterns.

Illumination

- Avoid positioning lighting fixtures directly over a bed; this will reduce the glare and spotlight effect in the individual's direct line of vision when lying on back.
- Design lighting to be indirect and diffused to reduce glare and shadow patterns (shadows sometimes appear to be dark holes or ghostlike figures).

Color

- Select a color scheme that includes warm hues and accents since cooler hues (such as blues) appear "washed out" to aged eyes.
- Use contrasting colors to distinguish rooms, door facings, furniture, etc.

Spatial Arrangement

- The dining room and bathroom should be clearly visible, accessible, and at a distance consistent with the individual's competency level.

Alzheimer patients who cannot directly see the bathroom are more likely to be incontinent. Whereas plumbing cannot readily be altered, a portable toilet may be used.

- Remove low-lying furniture (footstools, hassocks) from pathways to reduce risk of falls.

Pattern

- Avoid using sharp color contrasts in patterns displayed on wall coverings, floor coverings, window treatments, and upholstery materials. These patterns create visual complexity and can increase visual confusion.

- Avoid using abstract patterns that have strong color contrast and distorted designs.

Memory Impairment

The most common symptom of Alzheimer's disease is memory dysfunction. This impairment is exhibited in the individual through diminished decision-making skills, insecurity, and a loss of social skills. It also results in much confusion in interpreting visual and auditory information in the physical environment. There is difficulty understanding complexity in the environment, such as different colors and patterns, and in understanding the environment as a "whole"—that is, how individual components relate to the combined unit. In addition, the Alzheimer patient experiences reduced ability to determine size, color, and shape constancies. For example, when a person is far away, to our eye he is quite small, but we do not perceive the person to have become quite small; instead, his regular size remains constant in our perception. The inability to maintain constancies of perception can be confusing to an Alzheimer patient. The design elements to be considered with regard to these impairments are noise abatement/control, furnishings, spatial arrangement, pattern, and texture.

Noise Abatement/Control

- Monitor television programs to avoid movies and programs that include exploding bombs, gun shots, babies crying, and other sounds that can be confused with reality and can cause anxiety and negative behavioral acts such as screaming, crying, and hitting.

Furnishings

• Avoid using mirrors: they intensify anxiety when an individual no longer recognizes himself/herself.

• Recliners often become a hazard due to the mechanical operation required for reclining.

Spatial Arrangement

• Furniture arrangement on patios, in courtyards, and in sitting rooms should be grouped to encourage social interaction. Small groupings facilitate such interaction and reduce confusion due to noise and movements.

Pattern

• Avoid "still-life" patterns often found in floor coverings, wall coverings, window treatments, and upholstery materials; these can be confused with reality.

• Avoid floral wall coverings, floor coverings, and upholstery materials that often are thought to be "real" plant materials by the individual.

Texture

• Select soft textures that have a pleasant tactile quality.

• Avoid rough textures that are abrasive to the skin and the senses.

Physical Impairment

In addition to mental deficits associated with Alzheimer's disease, often the individual has a shuffling gait, poor posture, and uncoordinated body movements that result in clumsiness. The design elements of furnishings and spatial arrangement are to be considered if at least partial compensation is to be made for these deficits and to increase for the health, safety, and welfare of individuals.

Furnishings

• Table lamps should have a heavy, unbreakable base operable from one main switch.

• When using table lamps, place electrical cords where they cannot be stumbled over.

• Furniture components should be sturdy and noncollapsible (folding chairs and tables are not safe).

• Seating components need arms, high backs, and no low stretchers between front leg supports where feet or legs could get caught resulting in an injury or a fall.

• Chairs and sofas should not be too low or too soft, since rising from a chair may be difficult due to balance problems.

• All furniture components should have rounded or beveled edges on arm pieces.

• Bed mattresses can be placed on the floor for sleeping. (This is preferable to railed beds in which confused individuals may inadvertently injure themselves).

• Provide storage chests with large, deep drawers painted white on the inside and equipped with large hardware.

• Floor coverings should be firm, of a nonslip type, and should require low maintenance.

Spatial Arrangement

• Traffic areas should be free of low objects and small floor rugs or floor cloths.

• Avoid periodic rearranging of furniture components: this will make orientation difficult for the individuals and will increase the likelihood of stumbling or falling.

CONCLUSION

Creating a therapeutic environment for the Alzheimer patient is a complicated task for both caregivers and designers. A user-friendly approach in arriving at design solutions must be used in order to design living environments that meet the specific needs of the individuals who are cognitively and/or physically impaired. The design suggestions in this chapter are broadly stated to allow caregivers and designers creative latitude. Materials selection and color preferences should be determined by the designers and caregivers based on geographic location, the type of housing facility, codes and regulations, climate, topography, economic constraints, and future plans. These suggestions are not conclusive and much remains to be learned in this area. What may be the most important concept in designing is to attempt to perceive the world through the eyes and ears of an Alzheimer patient. Continue to think of ways to maintain familiarity, reduce confusion, and still provide a pleasant and appropriate living environment for these special individuals.

SUGGESTED READINGS

American Institute of Architects Foundation. *Design for Aging: An Architect's Guide.* Washington, D.C.: AIA Press, 1985.

Howell, S. C. *Designing for Aging.* Cambridge, Mass.: MIT Press, 1980.

Raschko, B. B. *Housing Interiors for the Disabled and Elderly.* New York: Van Nostrand Reinhold Company, 1987.

5

Specialized Nursing Care of the Alzheimer Patient

Esperanza V. Joyce and Kenn M. Kirksey

Providing nursing care to an Alzheimer patient involves attending to all aspects of the individual's life, much as would be done for a young child. The attending caregiver must insure a safe environment, adequate nutrition, maintenance of hygiene, adequate exercise, and a medical care plan. Of equal importance, the Alzheimer patient needs attention and affection in order to feel secure and loved.

Unlike caring for a child, the Alzheimer patient is fully grown. This larger size and heavier weight can make it more difficult to provide for the individual's needs. For example, changing the diaper of a two-hundred-pound man can be challenging.

One woman who was interviewed told about the time she spent two hours trying to get her husband out of the bathtub. She eventually had to call the fire department for help! Although she laughs about it now, it must have been far less humorous at the time.

Another woman laughs when she remembers trying to get her mother out of their small bathroom. When the mother blocked the daughter's exit, the daughter attempted to crawl between her mother's legs to get out of the bathroom. As she did so, her mother sat down and could not get back up. The mother rode "horsey" style until her daughter was able to crawl to a chair. This unusual event *points out that even the best caregiver cannot anticipate every eventuality. Nevertheless, some forethought and a sense of humor are useful in caring for an Alzheimer victim.*

In the following essay, Esperanza V. Joyce and Kenn M. Kirksey, both registered nurses, provide useful suggestions for safety, hygiene, elimination, nutrition, and communication.

As a humanistic profession, the primary concern of professional nursing is caring for people: it is based on knowledge derived from the biological, the physical, and the psychosocial sciences. Nurses must also understand that health and health behaviors are inseparable from culture. When dealing with patients from a different culture, nurses must be aware that responses to illness are determined by cultural beliefs and values. When in a practice setting, the professional nurse's aim is to determine the mental and physical needs of the patient and to initiate an independent plan of care that emphasizes patient and family teaching. In addition, nurses conduct preventive and rehabilitative nursing measures according to needs demonstrated by patients and families. This essay will share professional nurses' experiences in caring for Alzheimer patients.

The following case study is presented to illustrate nursing management of a hypothetical Alzheimer patient. Common symptoms and treatment strategies are described with the intention of providing practical information that might be used by caregivers.

Mr. Jones was a slender, seventy-year-old man who wore bifocals and walked with a cane. He began losing his memory four years ago. He would drive his car to town to get the mail or groceries, and by the time he got there, he had forgotten the original purpose for the trip. Mr. Jones had always been a good cardplayer and had played with his friends at the lodge for years. He reached the point where he couldn't remember how to play cards at all. The people around town observed how the widower was acting and such remarks as "Oh, he's just getting old and senile" were frequently heard. Mr. Jones's condition rapidly degenerated, and he would not leave the house at all. Neighbors brought his food and mail to him and helped him keep his house clean. He had always been a very happy person, but his friends noticed that he now seemed to be moody and depressed much of the time. When he was sixty-eight, he could no longer perform various tasks, such as cooking, that had been routine for him. He hired a live-in housekeeper, Ms. C., to help him with cooking, cleaning the house, and doing laundry. Ms. C. noticed that Mr. Jones was sometimes disoriented as to place and frequently disoriented as to time. He would tell her that he had enjoyed going to the "picture show," when actually he had only watched a movie on television. One night Ms. C. became alarmed when she got up at 2:00 A.M. to check on Mr. Jones and found that he was not in his bed.

She searched around the house and the yard. Mr. Jones was nowhere to be found. She called the police and a search was begun. Mr. Jones was found two hours later in the tall weeds of a vacant lot four blocks away. His face and arms were bruised and he had a deep laceration on his lip. He told the police he had fallen several times while he was out taking the dog for his usual 9:00 A.M. walk. The fact was that he didn't own a dog, and it was nighttime. Mr. Jones was taken to the emergency room and the laceration sutured. The physician recommended that he be admitted to the hospital for observation and tests. Test results showed that Mr. Jones had Alzheimer's disease.

SIGNS AND SYMPTOMS

In the early stages of Alzheimer's disease, the person is able to both perform self-care activities and function socially. Initially, changes in behavior may be subtle and infrequent. During this stage the person may deny the presence of any abnormality and may try to cover up his behavior with excuses. These changes are often attributed to other physical or mental problems. As time progresses the signs and symptoms become more frequent and are noticed by family and friends. The once quiet and friendly person may exhibit swings in mood and outbursts of anger. Tasks that were simple, such as cooking, playing cards, and driving a car, become difficult. There is difficulty concentrating, making decisions, and maintaining coordination.

As the disease advances, the person's attempts to cover up for the behavior become more difficult. Sleep may be interrupted and the person may experience hallucinations. In addition, safety becomes a concern because of restlessness and tendencies to wander off, especially at night.

The lack of ability to function independently is characteristic of the final stages of the disease. Profound weight loss, related to impaired intake of food and fluids, is sometimes noted. The activities of daily living, such as hygiene and elimination, can no longer be controlled. In addition, the inability to recognize self, family, and friends may contribute to feelings of anger and frustration.

SPECIALIZED NURSING CARE

During the assessment phase, the nurse collects information from the affected person, medical records, family, and other health professionals in order to formulate a nursing treatment plan. Information will be needed regarding the major concerns of the family, including when symptoms were first observed and discussion about the disease's progress. The nurse will gather information about any history of recent head trauma, viral illness, or other health-related disorders that might be associated with disorientation. Other areas to be assessed are: current medications, diet history, elimination patterns, recent memory loss, sleep disturbances, and mood changes. In addition, impairment of motor skills and changes in behavior, self-concept, self-esteem, and body image will be noted.

Following the assessment phase, treatment goals are formulated. The general goals related to Mr. Jones's care include: (1) maintaining an environment conducive to safety; (2) preventing injury to himself or others; (3) promoting comfort by providing a clean environment; (4) improving self-esteem through improved appearance; (5) maintaining adequate hygiene; (6) assuring physical and psychological comfort; (7) maintaining proper elimination of urine and feces; (8) maintaining nutritional balance and optimal weight; and (9) maintaining interactive communication and level of awareness.

Safety

Nursing plans emphasize the need to maintain an environment conducive to Mr. Jones's safety; therefore, Ms. C. is advised to lock up medications, forks, and knives that might cause injury. Ms. C. is also informed to lock doors when Mr. Jones is observed to be restless, to prevent him from wandering. Since Mr. Jones is left alone on occasion, access to matches and lighters is denied. He is provided with nonflammable clothing and, in order to prevent fire hazards, he is not allowed to wear loose sleeves near stove burners. Instructions are given to use plastic cups instead of glass and to use an electric shaver rather than razor blades that might cause injury. To reduce falls, rails are installed on walls near the toilet and the bathtub. Mr. Jones is provided with an identification bracelet in the event he becomes lost. The bracelet is also essential in the event of an emergency: it alerts authorities to his condition and assists in removing any suspicion of drug or alcohol intoxication. As Mr. Jones's disease progresses, the car keys are removed from his possession to prevent him from injuring himself or others.

Methods to Improve Safety

- Restrict or monitor use of matches and lighters.

- Do not allow loose sleeves to be worn near stove burners.

- Wear nonflammable clothing.

- When decreased sensation to pain or heat occurs, the caregiver should test bath water, observe the temperature of heating pads, and monitor the patient carefully if gas heaters are being used.

- Lower beds, raise siderails, turn night-light on.

- Provide sufficient lighting for stairs and hallways.

- Do not rearrange furniture and appliances, but keep them where the person is used to seeing them.

- Avoid slippery or irregular surfaces (floors, sidewalks, small rugs).

- Assist the person to go up or down stairs.

- Make sure shoes have support and are tied to prevent falls.

- Reduce clutter in rooms and on floors, tables, and closet shelves.

- Have the person use a cane when walking through crowds.

- Have the person wear an identification bracelet in case of an emergency.

- Remove keys to cars when person no longer is able to drive.

Hygiene

As Mr. Jones's level of understanding and his attention span decreased, it was important to assess self-care abilities. Was Mr. Jones able to bathe himself, properly clean himself after a bowel movement, brush his teeth, or dress himself? Since Mr. Jones's mental status was altered, Ms. C. needed to offer simple, direct, and concise instructions about how to perform these tasks when necessary. She was advised to break each task down into steps. For example, to brush the teeth: (1) get the toothpaste, (2) take the cap off, (3) place paste on the brush, and (4) then brush teeth. It was also important to allow adequate time to perform the tasks.

When dressing Mr. Jones or assisting him to dress himself, Ms. C.

was instructed to offer one item of clothing at a time. Loose-fitting clothing was suggested since it would make dressing easier. Another important consideration, resulting from Mr. Jones's unsteady gait, was to install a flexible hose shower nozzle that allowed him to sit while showering.

Methods to Improve Hygiene

- Make adjustments in bathroom area (i.e., hand bars, handrails, raised toilet seat, nonslip surfaces).
- Be simple, direct, and concise when speaking, so the person can follow directions.
- Break down tasks into steps.
- Allow time to perform tasks.
- When dressing the person, offer one item of clothing at a time. Loose fitting clothing is easier to put on.
- Include denture care and oral care in daily hygiene.

Elimination

Disorientation, impaired neurological functioning, and inability to locate the bathroom may create elimination problems for the Alzheimer patient. It is important to note changes in bowel habits, such as constipation or diarrhea, dribbling, or incontinence. It is also advisable to monitor fluid intake very carefully because of its effect on elimination.

Methods used to facilitate Mr. Jones's elimination included identifying the bathroom with a sign or a picture and providing adequate lighting at night to assist him in locating it. Mr. Jones was observed for restlessness and for other cues that indicate he might need to go to the bathroom; he was urged to go at frequent intervals (i.e., every four hours). He was encouraged to drink at least eight glasses of fluid during the daytime, but his fluid intake was limited before bedtime to reduce incontinence. Ms. C. was asked to look for swelling in his hands and feet. She was told to consult his doctor should this occur because it might mean he was retaining fluid.

To avoid constipation, laxatives or stool softeners were provided as needed. Since Mr. Jones wore adult diapers, because of urinary incontinence, the need to change them often was stressed, as was the need to apply lotion or powder to prevent skin breakdown.

Methods of Improving Elimination

- Identify the bathroom with a sign or a picture.

- Provide adequate lighting, especially at night, to assist in locating the bathroom.

- Encourage the person to go to the bathroom at frequent intervals (i.e., every four hours).

- Encourage drinking at least eight glasses of fluid during the daytime, but limit fluids before bedtime to prevent incontinence. Consult a doctor if swelling of feet and/or hands is noticed.

- Observe the patient for restlessness and other cues that he or she may need to go to the bathroom.

- Provide laxatives or stool softeners as appropriate to avoid constipation.

- If adult diapers are worn, they should be changed often and lotion or powder applied to prevent skin breakdown.

Nutrition

Like many Alzheimer patients, as Mr. Jones's disease progressed, alterations in nutrition were noticed: there was a significant weight loss. It became important to assess food likes and dislikes, to determine if he was able to feed himself, and to ascertain the nutritional value of the food he was eating. It was also important to determine if loose or missing teeth affected his nutrition. Ms. C. was advised to limit the number of choices that he could make, since his ability to decide was impaired. She was encouraged to give assistance with food selections as appropriate.

To further encourage adequate intake of calories, Mr. Jones was allowed sufficient time for meals, and privacy was provided so that he was not embarrassed by unacceptable eating habits. Finger food or foods that could be eaten with a spoon were provided because they were manageable and allowed him to be autonomous in his feeding. When Mr. Jones refused to eat adequately at mealtimes, small, frequent feedings were offered. Food supplements (such as Ensure) were used alternatively to assure proper nutrition.

Methods of Improving Nutrition

- Provide assistance with food selection as appropriate.

- Ensure privacy so the person is not embarrassed by unacceptable eating habits that may develop.

- When the patient refuses to eat regular food, consider using food supplements.

- Monitor the amount of fluids consumed.

- Offer frequent, small feedings.

- Limit the number of food choices, since decision-making is impaired.

- Since the patient's motor functioning has decreased, allow sufficient time for meals.

- Provide finger foods or foods that can be easily managed with a spoon.

- Allow the patient to be as autonomous as possible in feeding.

- Avoid extremely hot foods: guard against burns.

- Monitor weight at least once per week at the same time, preferably in the morning.

Communication

It proved helpful to listen attentively and to maintain eye contact while communicating with Mr. Jones. Approaching in a calm, pleasant manner, and speaking slowly and distinctly worked well to facilitate understanding. Ms. C. was advised to avoid confrontations when possible. Despite Mr. Jones's poor ability to communicate, it was very important that Ms. C. continue to spend time with Mr. Jones, talking with him and helping him feel related to others.

Methods to Improve Communication

- Speak slowly and distinctly.

- Approach in a calm and pleasant manner.

- Keep directions simple: use simple words and short sentences.

- Listen attentively and maintain eye contact.

- Offer appropriate praise when meaningful statements are made.

- Avoid confrontations.

- Select a time of day when the person is relaxed, then engage in conversation.

- Call the patient by name; often response is forthcoming when the first name is used, at least until the last stages of disease are reached.

- Provide objects to assist with orientation (i.e., clocks, calendars, etc.).

CONCLUSION

Caring for an Alzheimer patient presents a challenge to nurses and other caregivers. Even though it is often frustrating to care for persons with this disease, it is imperative to remember that they should be treated in a humane and caring manner, which preserves their dignity.

SUGGESTED READINGS

Barber, C. E., and Pasley, B. K. "Family Care of Alzheimer's Patients: The Role of Gender and Generational Relationship on Caregiver Outcomes." *Journal of Applied Gerontology* 14, no. 2 (June 1995): 172–92.

Clark, M. J. *Nursing in the Community,* 2d ed. East Norwalk, Conn.: Appleton and Lange, 1996.

Cox, C., and Monk, S. "Hispanic Culture and Family Care of Alzheimer's Patients." *Health and Social Work* 18, no. 2 (May 1993): 92–100.

Hanks, R. S. "The Limits of Care: A Case of Legal and Ethical Issues in Filial Responsibility." *Marriage and Family Review* 21, nos. 3–4 (1995): 239–57.

Jivanjee, P. "Enhancing the Well-being of Family Caregivers to Patients with Alzheimer's Disease." *Journal of Gerontological Social Work* 23, nos. 1–2 (1994): 31–48.

Kermis, M. D. *Mental Health in Late Life: The Adaptive Process.* Boston: Jones and Bontlett Publishers, Inc., 1986.

Lukovits, T. G., and McDaniel, K. D. "Behavioral Disturbance in Severe Alzheimer's Disease: A Comparison of Family Member and Nursing Staff

Reporting." *Journal of the American Geriatrics Society* 40, no. 9 (September 1992): 891–95.

Raffensperger, E. B., Zusy, M. L., and Marchesseault, L. C. *Clinical Nursing Handbook.* Philadelphia: J. B. Lippincott Company, 1986.

Thielman, J. "Minding My Father." *Men's Health* 10, no. 70 (September 1995): 98–103+.

6

Nutrition, Aging, and the Alzheimer Patient

Janice R. Hermann and Julian E. Spallholz

A mother and daughter were sitting in their lunchroom one afternoon when "Dad," who had Alzheimer's disease, entered from outside with a bird feather in his mouth. Mother and daughter looked at each other. "Where's the bird?!" asked the daughter.

Another Alzheimer family was having lunch at a Chinese restaurant. The family members were deep in conversation, and the husband ignored the frequent taps on his shoulder. He finally looked up just as his wife picked up an eggroll to throw at him. He successfully ducked the eggroll, but the people sitting at the next table were not so fortunate!

Good nutrition is important to the health and well-being of the Alzheimer patient. As suggested by the above stories, however, dining is more than just consuming an adequate number of calories. Eating is an important social activity. The sensitive caregiver feeds not only the body but the social being of the Alzheimer person by making mealtimes pleasant and entertaining experiences. In the following essay, nutritionists Janice R. Steward and Julian E. Spallholz discuss the needs of the Alzheimer patient and provide tips to overcome eating problems.

CHANGES IN NUTRITIONAL NEEDS WITH AGE

The nutritional needs of older adults are not much different from those of younger adults. However, the aging process gives each age group special characteristics. This is true for the older adult as well as for the teenager or the expectant mother. Some of the changes that occur with aging affect food intake and the body's use of food and nutrients. The major change in dietary recommendations for older adults is a decrease in the amount of calories needed. Nutritional needs for most vitamins and minerals remain about the same as one grows older. To get an adequate amount of vitamins and minerals in fewer calories requires careful meal planning.

Calories

Energy needs decline progressively throughout adult life as physical activity decreases and as the body's metabolism slows down. Consuming more calories than the body actually uses can result in weight gain. Excess weight increases your risk of developing many health problems. Some conditions associated with excess weight include high blood pressure, heart disease, stroke, adult onset diabetes, and certain cancers.

Calories come from fats, carbohydrates, protein, and alcohol. There are nine calories per gram of fat, and four calories per gram of carbohydrate and protein. Alcohol contains seven calories per gram. This means that for equal weights fats and alcohol have about twice the calories as carbohydrates and protein. Alcohol calories are sometimes called "empty calories" since alcohol provides no other nutritional benefits. The quickest way to decrease calories is to decrease the amount of fat eaten and/or alcohol consumed.

Increasing physical activity will also use more calories and can help in weight control. Walking is an effective exercise. Some other exercise activities include swimming, bowling, cycling, and dancing.

Protein

Protein needs remain approximately the same for individuals fifty-one years or older as for younger adults. Protein is needed to maintain healthy cells and to help build resistance to infection. Protein is also needed for wound healing and to make enzymes and hormones. The Recommended Dietary Allowance (RDA) for protein for persons fifty-one years or older is 63 grams for males and 50 grams for females. Two meat and two dairy servings each day will provide adequate protein. This is equal to approximately 6 ounces of meat and 2 cups of milk. Protein requirements can be affected by your health status. The added stress of injury or disease may increase protein needs.

Fat

Fat is a nutrient that gives us energy. Fats are the most concentrated source of food energy, providing nine calories per gram. Fat helps form cell membranes and carries the fat-soluble vitamins A, D, E, and K. Fat also provides the essential fatty acids that the body cannot make. Although fat is important in our diet, many adults eat more fat than they should. High-fat diets are considered a risk factor for heart disease, cancer, and obesity. By increasing the risk of obesity, high-fat diets may indirectly increase your risk of adult onset diabetes and high blood pressure.

The American Heart Association recommends that 30 percent or less of your calories come from fat. This is about 65 grams for a 2,000-calorie diet. When trying to lower fat in your diet don't omit meats and dairy products. These foods contribute to a well-balanced diet. Choose lean meats and low-fat dairy products, use low-fat preparation methods, and watch your portion size to reduce the fat content of these foods. Limit your use of added or hidden sources of fat that don't contribute nutrients to a well-balanced diet. Some examples are margarine, oils, salad dressings, chips, snack foods, and high-fat bakery items.

Carbohydrates

Carbohydrates provide energy for body cells and the central nervous system. There is no RDA for carbohydrates; however, it is recommended that 50 to 60 percent of calories come from carbohydrate-rich foods. Most should come from complex carbohydrate foods: cereals, grains, legumes, vegetables, and fruits. Consumption of simple carbohydrates or sugar-rich foods should be limited. Six or more servings of breads and cereals are recommended to provide adequate carbohydrates.

Many people think carbohydrate-rich foods are fattening. Actually the "fattening" part has usually been added. For example, a medium baked potato has approximately 80 calories. Adding 1 tablespoon of margarine and 2 tablespoons of sour cream adds approximately 225 calories for a grand total of 305 calories of which almost 75 percent are fat calories.

Vitamins and Minerals

Nutritional needs for most vitamins and minerals remain the same for older as for younger adults. Because older adults require fewer calories, it is important that foods selected are nutrient-rich and contribute to a well-balanced diet. To have a healthy diet, you must eat a variety of foods. Normally, a well-balanced diet using a variety of foods will provide adequate vitamins and minerals for any age. No single food can supply all nutrients in the amounts needed. Vegetables and fruits are important sources of vitamins A and C, folate, and fiber. Breads and cereals provide B vitamins, iron, and other minerals. Whole grain breads and cereals also supply fiber. Milk provides calcium, protein, riboflavin, and vitamins A and D. Meat, poultry, and fish provide protein, B vitamins, iron, zinc, and other minerals.

Dietary restrictions that are self-imposed can result in low intakes of certain vitamins and minerals. Most deficiencies among older adults involve vitamins and minerals associated with perishable fruits and vegetables, meat, and milk. These are foods often omitted from the diet due to cost, storage, long-term poor eating habits, difficulty in chewing, or poor appetite.

Water

Water is more critical to life than food. Lack of water will result in death sooner than will lack of food. The sensation of thirst tends to decline with age. As a result, despite the availability of fluids, many older adults become dehydrated. Adults need six to eight cups of water each day. Water can be taken in many forms such as water, fruit juice, milk, soups, coffee, tea, or soft drinks. Because caffeine acts as a diuretic and can cause fluid loss, decaffeinated beverages are recommended instead of caffeine beverages for fluid replacement.

Fiber

The many different types of fiber are divided into *soluble* and *insoluble* fibers. Both types of fiber are necessary for good health. Dietary fiber has been related to many health conditions. Fiber may be beneficial in cases of constipation, diarrhea, diverticulitis, cardiovascular disease, colon cancer, and diabetes. However, one should be cautious in assuming that dietary fiber is the only factor involved in these conditions.

The best way to increase fiber in the diet is from food sources. These sources include fruits, vegetables, whole grain breads and cereals, dried peas and beans, nuts, and seeds. Cooking, processing, and removing peels can reduce the fiber in foods. There is no Recommended Dietary Allowance for fiber. However, the American Cancer Institute recommends 20 to 30 grams of dietary fiber each day. It is important to check with your physician about fiber in your diet. Fiber intake may have to be modified in older adults who have problems with chewing, swallowing, or other medical conditions.

There are some tips to consider when increasing fiber in your diet. Increase fiber in your diet slowly. Increasing fiber too rapidly may cause unpleasant side effects such as bloating and gas. Since fiber absorbs water it is important to drink plenty of fluids when increasing dietary fiber. Too much dietary fiber can decrease mineral absorption. It is possible to get too much fiber with concentrated fiber supplements. Adequate dietary fiber can be obtained from foods without using fiber supplements.

Vitamin/Mineral Supplements

Vitamin and mineral supplements have their place in the medical treatment of certain nutrition-related diseases. However, growing older does not mean that you are unhealthy and need extra nutrients above those a varied diet can provide. Americans waste millions of dollars on vitamin and mineral supplements that they do not need. A well-chosen diet using a variety of foods can provide all needed nutrients. However, many older adults do not consume adequate diets. Other physical, psychological, and social factors can affect food intake of older adults, putting them at nutritional risk. Therefore, while it is possible to get all the nutrients for good health from food, many elderly are not able to do so.

While recommendations for routine nutrient supplements for all older adults is still debatable, taking megadoses (ten times the RDA) is clearly *unwarranted* without specific medical recommendations. One might think that more is better when taking nutrient supplements. However, a nutrient taken in concentrated amounts or in megadoses can be dangerous. It's easier to overdose with supplements than with food. Minerals in large amounts can be toxic, as can vitamins. The fat-soluble vitamins (vitamins A, D, E, and K) are stored in the body. Excessive doses of these vitamins can accumulate and be harmful. Dangerous levels can produce such symptoms as nausea, vomiting, and other serious side effects. Toxicity from water-soluble vitamins, such as vitamin C, is unlikely since excess amounts are flushed from the body in the urine. However, serious side effects can occur even with water-soluble vitamins. Because nutrients interact with each other, a balance of all nutrients is important. If the body has too much or too little of any nutrient, the body's use of these nutrients may be altered.

Supplements are required to have the RDA and the percent (%) of the RDA on the label. If a single dose supplies 100 percent or less of the RDA, then a single dose is enough to ensure dietary adequacy. But, if the dose supplies 900 percent of the RDA, then that dose is nearing the mega-dose level and should be avoided. Additional supplements should *never* be used to replace a missed meal. You can not rely on a supplement to balance a poor diet. In fact, no supplement contains all the essential nutrients your body needs. The basis for good health depends on an adequate diet containing a variety of foods which supply sufficient amounts of calories and nutrients.

NUTRITION AND ALZHEIMER'S DISEASE: CAUSE AND EFFECT?

As Dr. Hutton discussed in his treatment of the medical aspects of dementia (see chapter 2), there presently is no single known cause or any associations of lifetime events that lead to the specific type of dementia known as Alzheimer's disease. There are only theories suggesting cause-and-effect relationships, which provide some direction for future research. Since we are what we eat, a legitimate question is: "Does diet alone, in any way, contribute to the onset of Alzheimer's disease?" The answer to this question is most certainly no. It is possible; however, that some dietary components of food, over which we have no control, may participate in the disease once it has begun.

The most studied dietary component observed to be associated with Alzheimer's disease is aluminum. It seems clear that aluminum does not cause Alzheimer's disease. After all, many people use aluminum cookware, and we store foods in aluminum containers. Aluminum is a major component of numerous antacids and deodorants, and many foods naturally contain aluminum. The mineral is also abundant in the soil, normally nontoxic, and has no known nutrition function. Aluminum accumulates in the brain plaques of Alzheimer patients as the disease progresses. The concentration of two other minerals, silicon and calcium, have also been observed to be concentrated in the brain plaques. Bromine and nickel, two more nonessential dietary components, have been found to be elevated in the blood and spinal fluid of a small sampling of Alzheimer patients.

While the source of these minerals is probably dietary, at this time the evidence is insufficient to conclude that common dietary practices contribute to the onset of Alzheimer's disease.

NUTRITIONAL NEEDS AND THE ALZHEIMER PATIENT

Once a patient is suspected of having Alzheimer's disease, comprehensive physical, radiological, and neuropsychological examinations will likely be performed by the attending physician. A full nutritional assessment may also be warranted at this time. Since Alzheimer's disease is a slow, progressive illness, many patients will at first appear in excellent physical health. Severe dementia brought on by nutritional imbalances or deficiencies is rare, but some instances of mental impairment among persons over the age of sixty have been associated with lower-than-average vitamin intake or an inability to utilize certain vitamins. A physical examination and nutritional assessment will likely exclude the possibility that the dementia has a dietary origin.

The gradual mental decline usually associated with Alzheimer's disease is typically accompanied by physical decline of the patient. Such decline is the combined result of neuromuscular impairment, a reduction in ability to exercise, and inadequate nutritional intake. Confusion, gradual loss of short-term recall, and a shortened attention span may result in the Alzheimer patient not completing or even skipping meals. Selecting the proper eating utensil may become a difficult and frustrating mental task. The caregiver will eventually have to make what appear to be simple decisions for the Alzheimer patient.

Meals skipped, excessive irritability, and reduced sleeping hours over extended periods of time may place the Alzheimer patient in a continual negative calorie condition. Under such eating conditions, protein-calorie malnutrition may occur, and the patient will begin to lose weight. It seems reasonable, therefore, that attention to the patient's weight and caloric intake are the first defenses that a family can take against the physical deterioration associated with Alzheimer's disease.

Reduced caloric intake and weight loss lead to reductions in both vitamin and mineral intake, even if smaller amounts of a balanced diet are eaten by the patient. Protein-calorie malnutrition hastens vitamin/mineral deficiencies unless a vitamin/mineral supplement is provided. However, there are no data suggesting that vitamin/mineral supplements either retard or accelerate the course of Alzheimer's disease. Caregivers should consult with the attending physician concerning use of a vitamin/mineral supplement.

Protein-calorie malnutrition is frequently encountered in elderly patients in hospitals and other institutional settings as a condition secondary to the primary disease. Inadequate food intake frequently arises from mental decline, loss of physical dexterity, difficulty in swallowing, and the need to be spoon-fed by a caregiver. Without necessary caloric intake, vitamin/mineral deficiency can lead to impairment of the immune system or the blood. The immune system is responsible for combating infectious disease, including pneumonia, which occurs frequently in Alzheimer's patients. Impairment of the blood system may result in anemia, thereby further weakening the patient.

During the advanced stages of Alzheimer's disease, the patient's family may be confronted with the decision to provide nutritional support therapy by nasogastric tube or total parenteral nutrition (TPN), administered through a tube into the esophagus or stomach. Such decisions, often difficult to make, usually reside with family members after consultation with the attending physician.

Protein-calorie malnutrition associated with vitamin/mineral deficiencies and dehydration are frequent consequences of Alzheimer's disease. Vitamin-mineral deficiencies are readily preventable through the course of the disease by providing solid or liquid supplements. Dehydration can be prevented by noting sufficient consumption of liquids. Protein-calorie malnutrition is more difficult to prevent. Increased family awareness of nutritional aspects, professional assistance, and more attention to the nutritional management of the Alzheimer patient may slow the rate of mental and physical decline of the Alzheimer patient.

TIPS TO HELP MAINTAIN FOOD INTAKE

Consuming an adequate diet is necessary to obtain nutrients and to help individuals stay healthy. The following tips are suggestions that have worked for some Alzheimer patients. However, each patient is different; the caregiver will need to determine what may work for a particular patient. Caregivers need to understand the progressive nature of this disease; solutions that work today may not necessarily work in the future.

Many of the physical, emotional, and social changes that occur with aging can cause may people to lose their appetite as they grow older. Not all of these problems can be corrected, but interest in eating a well-balanced nutritious diet must be maintained. Nutritional needs do not decrease as individuals grow older, except for a reduction in the amount of calories needed. A well-balanced nutritious diet can be the best defense an individual has for staying healthy and preventing illness. The following suggestions may help increase interest and food intake for older persons who have decrease in appetites.

Tips to Increase Appetite:

- Have the main meal of the day at breakfast or lunch when appetite is larger, keeping the dinner meal smaller.

- Have five or six smaller meals, rather than only two or three larger meals.

- Take a daily walk or have other physical activity to increase appetite.

- Use familiar foods fixed in a familiar way.

- If the patient simply refuses to eat a balanced diet or is not consuming enough calories, consult with the attending physician about using vitamin and/or mineral supplements.

- Try to include at least one food item in the meal you know the patient likes.

Tips to Overcome Mealtime Confusion

- Make mealtime a routine that occurs at the same time, in the same place, and with as little confusion as possible.

- Make sure physical surroundings are pleasant and calm, avoiding unnecessary distractions.

- Set aside ample time for meals so they are not rushed.

- Serving one food item at a time may result in less confusion.

Tips to Overcome Eating Problems

- When a patient clenches his/her teeth, spits out food, becomes unruly, or demonstrates other disruptive eating behaviors, try discontinuing mealtime for a few minutes. Taking a short break can be helpful to both the patient and the caregiver. Sometimes just having a different person feed a patient can be helpful.

- Be alert to the patient while feeding. A patient may spit out food not because he/she is being difficult, but because he/she is having a difficult time eating. Do not continue to feed a patient if he/she appears to be choking or coughing.

- Have meals in complete privacy if the patient is embarrassed about his/her inability to feed himself/herself.

- A patient may not have the judgment to know what should and should not be eaten; the caregiver may have to make those decisions. This is particularly important regarding special diets or when removing non-nutritive foods such as salt, ketchup, or seasonings that should not be consumed in excess.

- When messiness or spills become a problem due to loss of coordination, there are many steps that can be taken to adjust.

  - Try using plastic tablecloths and a plastic apron for the patient; this will ease the cleaning-up process.

  - Plastic plates and cups are easier to handle and less likely to break than glass or pottery. Plastic utensils, however, can break easily and may be dangerous.

  - Utensils with large built-up handles can be held more easily. Foam handles can be built so that utensils are easier to grip.

  - There are many specially designed dishes and utensils available at medical supply stores that can make eating easier.

  - CAUTION HOT! Mugs with lids can prevent spills but can be dangerous. Hot beverages are much hotter if consumed through a straw or from a mug with a lid that only has a small opening for the liquid, and can cause serious burns.

- There are meal programs available, such as "Meals-on-Wheels" or "Congregate Meal Programs," that can assist by delivering meals to the home.

**Tips to Increase Food Intake if
Chewing and Swallowing Are Problems**

• Be sure dentures fit properly.

• Use gravy or sauces to help moisten food.

• Provide fluids at mealtime to help with swallowing. If fluids such as water are difficult to swallow, try Jell-O or milkshakes.

• Encourage the patient to eat slowly and chew food thoroughly. Verbal reminders may be needed.

• If the patient is not able to chew regular meats, use soft meat alternatives to maintain adequate protein intake. Foods such as deviled eggs, egg salad, soft meat salads, meat soups or milk-based soups, milk pudding, and custards are suitable substitutions.

• Try mashing or shredding foods. Using shredded fruits or vegetables in salads, Jell-O, or stir-fry may increase food intake.

• Avoid grinding food: it becomes dry and difficult to swallow unless broth or gravy is used to help moisten the food. It is better to maintain as normal a dietary pattern as possible. Try precutting foods and putting the smaller bite-size pieces into casseroles and soups so that the food is easier to eat but the patient still feels he/she is eating regular foods.

• Avoid using baby foods if possible. If a pureed diet is necessary, try using a blender or food grinder to puree normally prepared foods. Using baby foods may unknowingly be degrading to the patient, thus making him/her feel as if he/she is being treated like a child.

Tips to Increase Food Intake if Taste and Smell Decline

• If taste sensation has diminished, try using foods that vary in texture and temperature.

• Enhancing the flavors of foods with spices can increase the acceptance of foods by those patients whose taste acuity has decreased.

• The sense of different tastes (sweet, salt, bitter) are best perceived at body temperature. Patients will be more aware of different flavors if food is served at body temperature (rather than normal serving temperatures).

- Serve colorful and attractive foods. Foods taste better if they are attractive.

- Along with a decline in taste and smell, the Alzheimer patient may not be able to determine the temperature of food or beverages. Therefore, check the temperature (especially for beverages) before serving This practice will avoid burns.

CONCLUSION

Though proper nutrition will not cure Alzheimer's disease, it is nevertheless vital to the patient's well-being and may help to prevent the onset of other complications including malnutrition and pneumonia. Caregivers should be aware that medications may interfere with the absorption or utilization of nutrients and, over prolonged periods of time, could lead to some nutritional deficiencies. The advice of a physician or pharmacist may be needed concerning possible drug/nutrient interactions.

We must also remember that although the patient is in a demented state, he or she may at times be perfectly lucid. The patient should always be treated with dignity, respect, and concern for individual self-worth.

A useful way to remember nutritional support for Alzheimer patients is "MEALTIMES":

M — Maintain a routine
E — Eat well-balanced meals
A — Alertness to any nutritional problems
L — Light and frequent meals
T — Teach the caregiver how to deal with the patient
I — Interactions between drugs and nutrients
M — Minimize confusion for the patient
E — Encourage patient to eat
S — Supplement the diet when necessary

APPENDIX
FOOD GUIDE PYRAMID: A GUIDE TO DAILY FOOD CHOICES

The most useful guide currently available for food selection is the Food Guide Pyramid. The Food Guide Pyramid puts the dietary guidelines into

Food Guide Pyramid

A Guide to Daily Food Choices

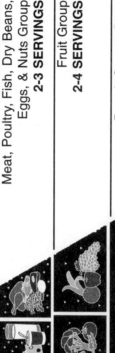

KEY

○ Fat (naturally occurring and added)

▽ Sugars (added)

These symbols show that fat and added sugars come mostly from fats, oils, and sweets, but can be part of or added to foods from the other food groups as well.

Fats, Oils, & Sweets
USE SPARINGLY

Milk, Yogurt, & Cheese Group
2-3 SERVINGS

Meat, Poultry, Fish, Dry Beans, Eggs, & Nuts Group
2-3 SERVINGS

Vegetable Group
3-5 SERVINGS

Fruit Group
2-4 SERVINGS

Bread, Cereal, Rice, & Pasta Group
6-11 SERVINGS

Use the Food Guide Pyramid to help you eat better every day . . . the Dietary Guidelines way. Start with plenty of Breads, Cereals, Rice, and Pasta; Vegetables; and Fruits. Add two to three servings from the Milk group and two to three servings from the Meat group. Each of these food groups provides some, but not all, of the nutrients you need. No one food group is more important than another—for good health you need them all. Go easy on fats, oils, and sweets, the foods in the small tip of the Pyramid.

action. The pyramid is an outline of what to eat each day. It is not a rigid prescription, but a general guide that lets you choose a healthy diet. The pyramid calls for eating a variety of foods to get the nutrients you need.

Looking At the Pieces of the Pyramid

The Food Guide Pyramid emphasizes foods from five major food groups. Each of these food groups provides some, but not all, of the nutrients you need every day. Foods in one group can't replace another. No one food group is more important than another; for good health you need them all.

Bread, Cereal, Rice, and Pasta Group

Breads, cereals, rice, and pasta are all foods from grains. You need the most servings of these foods each day. These foods are important because they provide complex carbohydrates. Complex carbohydrates are an important source of energy, especially in low-fat diets. They also provide B vitamins, protein, iron, fiber, and other trace minerals. The Food Guide Pyramid suggests **6 to 11** servings each day. One serving is any of the following:

> 1 slice of bread
> $\frac{1}{2}$ hamburger or hot dog bun
> 1 ounce of ready-to-eat cereal
> $\frac{1}{2}$ cup of cooked rice or pasta
> $\frac{1}{2}$ cup of cooked cereal

Vegetable Group

Vegetables are important because they provide vitamins such as A and C, and folate. They also provide minerals such as iron and magnesium. Vegetables are naturally low in fat and are good sources of fiber. The Food Guide Pyramid suggests **3 to 5** servings each day. One serving is any of the following:

> 1 cup of raw leafy vegetables
> $\frac{1}{2}$ cup of chopped raw or cooked vegetables
> $\frac{3}{4}$ cup of vegetable juice

Fruit Group

Fruits and fruit juices provide important amounts of vitamin C and potassium. Fruits are naturally low in fat and sodium, and are also good sources of fiber. The Food Guide Pyramid suggests **2 to 4** servings each day. One serving is any of the following:

1 medium apple, banana, orange, pear, or peach
$\frac{1}{2}$ cup of chopped, cooked, or canned fruit
$\frac{1}{4}$ cup of dried fruit
$\frac{3}{4}$ cup of fruit juice

Milk, Yogurt, and Cheese Group

The milk, yogurt, and cheese group provides calcium, protein, phosphorus, and vitamins A, D, B_6, and B_{12}. Dairy products are your best food source of calcium. The Food Guide Pyramid suggests **2** servings each day for most people. One serving is any of the following:

1 cup milk or yogurt
$1\frac{1}{2}$ ounces of natural cheese
2 ounces of processed cheese

Meat, Poultry, Fish, Beans, Eggs, and Nut Group

Meat, poultry, and fish supply protein, iron, zinc, and vitamins B_6 and B_{12}. The other foods in this group—dry beans, eggs, and nuts—are similar to meats in providing protein and most minerals. The Food Guide Pyramid suggests **2 to 3** servings each day of foods from this group. The total amount of these servings should be the equivalent of 5 to 7 ounces of cooked lean meat, poultry, or fish per day. One serving is any of the following:

2 to 3 ounces of cooked lean meat, poultry, or fish. Three ounces is about the size of a deck of playing cards.
$\frac{1}{2}$ cup of cooked beans, 1 egg, or 2 tablespoons of peanut butter is 1 ounce of lean meat, or about $\frac{1}{3}$ serving.

Fats and Sugars

At the tip of the pyramid are fats, oils, and sweets. These are foods such as salad dressings, oils, cream, butter, margarine, sugars, soft drinks, candies, and sweet desserts. These foods provide calories but few nutrients.

The small circles in the pyramid symbolize the fat content in foods. The small triangles in the pyramid symbolize the sugar content of foods. The fat and sugar symbols are concentrated in the tip of the pyramid, but some fat or sugar symbols are shown in the other food groups. This is because some food choices in the food groups can also be high in fat or added sugars.

How Many Servings Are Right for You?

The pyramid shows a range of servings for each food group. The number of servings that is right for you depends on how many calories you need. The following table shows the suggested number of servings at different calorie levels.

Suggested Number of Servings at Three Calorie Levels

	1,600 calories	2,200 calories	2,800 calories
Bread Group	6 servings	9 servings	11 servings
Vegetable Group	3 servings	4 servings	5 servings
Fruit Group	2 servings	3 servings	4 servings
Milk Group	2–3 servings	2–3 servings	2–3 servings
Meat Group (oz.)	5 servings	6 servings	7 servings

For additional nutrition information, contact thse organizations:

National: Alzheimer's Association
919 N. Michigan Ave.
Suite 1000
Chicago, IL 69611
1–800–621–9379

State: Contact the Cooperative Extension Service nutrition specialist located at your state's Land Grant University or your county Cooperative Extension Service office.

Local: Contact the local United Way Agency, Dietetic Association, or local Alzheimer's chapter. The national Alzheimer's Association can provide information on your local Alzheimer's chapter.

SUGGESTED READINGS

Mace, N. L., and Rabins, P. V. *The Thirty-Six Hour Day.* Baltimore: Johns Hopkins University Press, 1991.

Schlenker, E. D. *Nutrition in Aging,* 2d ed. St. Louis: Mosby-Year Book, Inc., 1993.

Zarit, S. H., Orr, N. K., and Zarit, J. M. *The Hidden Victims of Alzheimer's Disease: Families Under Stress.* New York: New York University Press, 1985.

7

Speech and Hearing Deficits Associated with Alzheimer's Disease

Roger F. Clem

A lack of good judgment and problems with language and communication are hallmarks of Alzheimer's disease. Attempts to ascertain the true level of competence of an Alzheimer patient is sometimes a difficult task, as one Texas judge learned.

The elderly Alzheimer patient, Mr. T., was sitting in his wheelchair in front of a store, waiting for his wife to make a purchase, when he was robbed. Fortunately the thief was caught and brought to trial. During the trial, the judge asked Mr. T. if he had given the accused his wallet, as this was the defense that the accused had offered. Mr. T. looked long and hard at the judge before replying, "That's a damn stupid question!" In this case, Mr. T. clearly understood the question and communicated his response quite well, but his judgment might be questioned!

In the essay that follows, Roger F. Clem, an audiologist, briefly describes the language and communication deficits that may be expected to develop during the course of Alzheimer's disease. The art in caring for an Alzheimer patient is to not underestimate the true capacity of the patient to comprehend and to communicate. To do so robs the individual of remaining competence. At the same time, to overestimate the true capacity will lead to frustration on the part of both the caregiver and the patient.

Most individuals will experience some type of communication problem during the aging process. As a person ages, a number of natural changes occur that reduce sensory acuity. This gives rise to less precise communication. After the age of sixty, individuals generally see and hear less well than in their youth. Sensory decline is expected with age and not considered abnormal unless such deficits are major. For example, while a certain amount of hearing loss is considered normal as one grows older, acquired deafness is not considered a normal factor accompanying old age. Also, it is not unusual to wear glasses (or require bifocals) as one ages, but total loss of sight is abnormal.

COMMUNICATION

People with Alzheimer's disease have many problems communicating with others. Although these communication problems involve some deficits in their speech and language, it is not possible to discuss speech or hearing problems as they relate to communication without also examining the relationship between speech/hearing and language.

Physiologically, speech can be considered the result of the appropriate use of the lips, tongue, teeth, and vocal cords to produce sounds. The pure mechanics of speech (making speech sounds) can be accomplished without imparting any information to the listener, especially if the speech sounds have no meaning. Choosing the desired words and ordering them in a fashion that will accomplish the intended meaning involves language. The symbols that are used during oral communication are words. Even if all of the words of a sentence are produced clearly and concisely, no meaning can be derived if the sentence is not organized in a logical fashion with words that conform to the speaker's intended mental image.

In much the same way, hearing involves not only the basic reception of sounds but also the processing of these acoustical items in a fashion that matches the perceptions with meaningful information in the brain. It is quite possible for a person to hear everything that is spoken on a pure awareness or sensory basis but not derive any meaning or symbol association from these sounds. Therefore, the comprehension and understanding of a spoken message is equally dependent on not only the awareness of all of the acoustical elements of what was spoken, but also the mental organization of the speech sounds and the brain's association of these sounds with meaningful linguistic symbols. For example, a person might hear every component of a message that is being presented in Chinese but be unable to understand what is said. The person's hearing acuity is adequate to perceive all of the components of the message, but no association can be made between the auditory perception and any meaningful information.

Effective communication must involve both a speaker's articulation and the hearing of the listener. The speaker must produce the words correctly and organize them in an appropriate fashion. The listener must be able to hear all of the components of the spoken message and be able to associate meaning with what is heard.

SPEECH AND LANGUAGE PROBLEMS IN ALZHEIMER'S DISEASE

The normal aging process does not create major deficits in the intelligibility or the appropriate organization of speech. However, those persons who are afflicted with Alzheimer's disease are atypical because they undergo brain changes in areas that appear to be highly associated with memory and language. The mechanical components of speech production remain relatively unaffected by Alzheimer's disease until the final stages of the disorder. It is disturbance in the meaningfulness of language that is most pronounced throughout the progression of the disease.

The major aspects of disrupted communication arising in Alzheimer's disease are language problems that result from cognitive decline. One of the first problems to occur involves the forgetting of appropriate words or the use of "pseudowords" in place of the forgotten item. For example, a person might use the term *pencicle* to describe a ballpoint pen, or the term *firebugs* to describe matches. There is also difficulty naming objects, particularly specific names. The Alzheimer patient, for example, may be able to identify a picture as that of a dog, but not as that of a "collie," which is a higher order name. The communication problem is not one of articulation but a deficit in generating the appropriate words with which to convey information on a symbolic level.

The Alzheimer patient is generally unaware of these communication problems; his/her speech is frequently characterized by an empty, aimless quality. Much of this pointless vocalization is the result of verbal wandering characterized by repetitive speech with little comprehensible meaning. The spoken words are produced correctly and with appropriate fluency but with limited ability to communicate meaningfully.

As the disease progresses, problems will occur in generating words, naming objects, and recognizing meaningful relationships. For example, forks, knives, and spoons may no longer have a relationship to one another for a person experiencing the symptoms of Alzheimer's disease. He or she may begin to engage in *echolalia,* repeating the same word or phrase over and over. These verbal repetitions will occur with little or no comprehension of what was said. Echolalia may progress to the point where vocalizing deteriorates to repetitious syllables that are unrecognizable as language.

With Alzheimer's disease there is also a decreased ability to recognize some of the pragmatic aspects of speech. *Pragmatics* involve the rules of speech and language as they apply to usage. Adjusting one's rhetoric to suit the audience, not standing too close to the listener, and using body language to help convey intentions are all part of the pragmatics of communication. Other examples of pragmatics include asking questions by using the appropriate inflection, or greater emphasis being placed on certain statements by the way words are spaced and timed. Lacking awareness of the pragmatics of a certain situation, a person might not respond in the desired or appropriate manner.

In advanced stages of Alzheimer's disease communication has progressed to such an extent that the individual is essentially mute. Spontaneous speech may all but cease, and echolalic behavior is quite common. At this point the patient may have difficulty even with the physical generation of speech sounds.

HEARING IMPAIRMENT

One of the expected changes that occur during normal aging is a decrease in hearing acuity. The term used for hearing loss associated with the aging process is *presbycusis.* This impairment is the product of many factors having to do with what the individual's condition and the environment to which he or she has been exposed. Some contributing factors include noise exposure, toxic substances, hypertension, vascular insufficiency, and anatomical changes in the hearing system. In reality, presbycusis relates to numerous disorders under the category of hearing loss resulting from the aging process.

The average person affected by Alzheimer's disease will also experience presbycusis. Therefore, it is to be expected that the individual will develop some high-frequency hearing difficulty and problems in understanding speech. Those with high-frequency hearing loss will have numerous problems understanding when in noisy situations. Therefore, when talking to a person who has Alzheimer's disease it is always wise to select a quiet environment and reduce the rate of speaking to allow greater time for the patient to understand what is spoken.

SPEECH AND HEARING SERVICES

Individuals with Alzheimer's disease experience communication problems that are language-based, rather than a function of peripheral disorders (i.e., damage to the ear). This inability to communicate effectively is a symptom of the underlying brain impairment. Speech, language, and hearing therapy can do nothing to arrest these underlying neurological problems, and traditional ways of treating speech and language deficits are ineffective for Alzheimer patients (see chapter 9). Ways exist to increase communication through gestural techniques that will greatly aid in both the physical and emotional care of these patients.

Hearing impairment of a magnitude sufficient to create communication problems commonly exist with the Alzheimer patient. Unfortunately, the cognitive impairment associated with the dementia may preclude the proper use of hearing aids in the later stages of the illness. If hearing impairment is a suspected factor in communication problems, particularly in the early stages of Alzheimer disease, then an audiological referral might be considered. Because hearing impairment is a normal factor in the aging process, routine audiological evaluations are a wise precaution for all older persons. The present state of technological advancement in the design and use of hearing aids can now provide assistance to people with types of hearing impairment that could not have been satisfactorily fitted with amplification even five years ago.

If speech, language, or hearing services are desired one of the best resources is the phone book. The yellow pages, under speech and hearing services, speech pathology, speech therapy, audiology, and hearing testing, list a number of professionals and businesses that provide these services. When dealing with an audiologist or speech-language-pathologist, it is important to note if the professional has a Certificate of Clinical Competence (CCC) from the American Speech-Language-Hearing Association (ASHA). A CCC in either speech pathology or audiology indicates that the individual has obtained a Masters degree or its equivalent in that field, has served an apprentice period under qualified supervision, and has passed a national qualifying examination in the discipline.

The American Speech-Language-Hearing Association is another fine resource in obtaining information and direction concerning speech and hearing problems. The consumer division of ASHA, or the National Association of Hearing and Speech Action (NAHSA), can be contacted at 10801 Rockville Pike, Rockville, Maryland 20852, or by telephone at 1-800-638-TALK. Those who are curious about hearing impairment can contact NAHSA, which will then mail a list of all ASHA recognized speech and/or hearing centers within a particular state or mail packets of information concerning hearing impairment to the interested party.

SUGGESTED READINGS

Appel, J., and Kertsz, A. "A Study of Language Functioning in Alzheimer Patients." *Brain and Language* 17 (1982): 73–91.

Cummings, J. L., and Benson, D. F. *Dementia. A Clinical Approach.* Boston: Butterworths, 1983.

Darby, J. K. (ed.). *Speech and Language Evaluation in Neurology: Adult Disorders.* New York: Harcourt Brace Jovanovich, 1985.

Grimes, A. M., Grady, C. L., Foster, N. L., Sunderland, T., Patronas, N. J., et al. "Central Auditory Function in Alzheimer's Disease." *Neurology* 35 (1985): 352–58.

Johns, D. F. (ed.). *Clinical Management of Neurogenic Communicative Disorders.* Boston: Little, Brown and Company, 1985.

Reisberg, B. *A Guide to Alzheimer's Disease.* New York: Macmillan, Inc., 1981.

Sacks, O. W. *The Man Who Mistook His Wife for a Hat.* New York: Summit Books, 1985.

Schwartz, M. F., Marin, O. S. M., and Saffran, E. M. "Dissociation of Language Function in Dementia: A Case Study." *Brain and Language* 7 (1979): 277–306.

Ulatowska, H. K. *The Aging Brain: Communication in the Elderly.* San Diego: College-Hill Press, 1985.

8

Memory and Language Deficits
in Alzheimer's Disease

David B. Mitchell, Ph.D.

Everyone has lapses in memory from time to time. Remember the time that you forgot to cut the price tags off of your clothes before you wore them, or forgot to send your wife flowers on your anniversary? We frequently find humor in stories about times in our lives when memory failed us. Such anecdotes arise even for the families of Alzheimer patients. One of our favorite stories is about a woman who, though in the early stages of Alzheimer's disease, had been unwittingly selected to serve as a juror in a murder trial. One day, about midway through the trial, the jurors were excused for their lunch break. Much to the court's dismay, the woman forgot *to come back, and the judge had to declare a mistrial!*

Despite the belief that memory declines sharply with age, this is not actually what occurs. David B. Mitchell, a developmental psychologist, discusses the differences in memory and language that occur with age, as compared to those that take place with Alzheimer's disease. He explains how some components of memory are lost before others. By understanding the thinking processes of Alzheimer patients, we may better facilitate their adaptation and may decrease our own sense of frustration.

Consider these words: *dinosaur, avocado, tequila.* We'll come back to them later.

Alzheimer's disease is often described by professionals as a disorder of memory and cognition (thought processes). Indeed, memory loss is usually the first symptom that the individual or the spouse notices and brings to the attention of the family physician. Difficulty recalling names of familiar places and objects is commonly reported, as well as problems remembering where objects were placed. Other language problems, related to vocabulary, can also appear early, and are virtually inevitable as the disease progresses.

A number of assessment scales are now available, both for more thorough diagnosis and for plotting the severity of the disease. Thomas Hutton and his colleagues have developed the Functional Rating Scale, which assesses a variety of everyday behaviors including eating, dressing, speech, memory, degree of confusion, orientation, emotionality, social responsiveness, and sleep patterns (see chapter 2). Barry Reisberg has developed Functional Assessment Stages (FAST), and there is a Record of Independent Living (RIL) scale to assess day-to-day functional competence. In recent research, a strong relationship has been found between these functional scales and clinical scales such as the Dementia Rating Scale and the Global Deterioration Scale. These scales are also useful for plotting and predicting stages of functional decline in patients in long-term care settings.

For example, the *mild cognitive decline* stage in the Global Deterioration Scale, developed by Barry Reisberg and colleagues, is characterized by a level of impaired functioning noticeable to co-workers and difficulty traveling to new places. In the *moderate decline* or *late confusional* stage, individuals will often fail in attempting to carry out relatively complex tasks such as planning meals and handling their finances. Individuals in the *moderately severe* stage require assistance in *choosing* proper clothing, while those in the *severe stage* have trouble just putting their clothes *on*. In the very late stages of the disease, patients lose all memory and language abilities (including recollection of their spouse's name), basic motor skills (such as walking), and bladder control. Since memory and language function are nonexistent in the late stages of dementia, the remainder of this chapter will focus on the mild to moderate stages.

MULTIPLE MEMORY SYSTEMS

When patients have memory complaints or when professionals discuss memory loss, it is often assumed that memory is a singular trait. In fact, however, there is increasing evidence for several types of memory. The distinction between different memory systems is important because some systems may be affected by aging or by disease, while other systems may remain intact. At least three types of long-term memory representation (conceived by Endel Tulving at the University of Toronto) are important for understanding the differential effects of normal aging versus disease: episodic memory, semantic memory, and implicit memory.

Episodic (or event) *memory* involves conscious recollection of specific events in your life that occurred in a particular time and place. What were you doing when you heard that John Kennedy was assassinated? When the space shuttle *Challenger* exploded after liftoff? Where did you spend Thanksgiving last year? When did you last see your spouse? What did you eat for breakfast today? All of these remembrances require episodic memory, which allows us (sometimes!) to remember *what, when,* and *where.* Note that episodic memory contains information ranging from a few minutes ago to many years ago. (*Short-term* or *Working Memory*—which serves our moment-to-moment conscious thinking—is a category separate from the long-term memory systems under discussion.)

Semantic memory contains our vocabulary and general knowledge of the world, information that is available independent of time and context. Who was John Kennedy? What do you usually eat for Thanksgiving? What kinds of clothes should you wear to your nephew's wedding? What is your spouse's name? Note the difference between these questions and the episodic memory questions in the previous paragraph. In the memory laboratory, we might ask someone to name some fruits (semantic memory) or to recall the names of some fruits from a list presented earlier (episodic memory). Healthy older adults—compared to young adults—do experience greater difficulty with episodic memory, but not with semantic memory. Alternatively, patients suffering from Alzheimer's disease suffer loss of both types of memory.

Implicit (or procedural) *memory* is the most basic type of memory, as it simply requires a response in the presence of a previously experienced stimulus. At the piano or computer keyboard, our fingers seem to "know" where the keys are. When a traffic light turns red, our right foot goes automatically to the brake pedal. When we see a familiar printed word, its pronunciation is immediately available. The second time we visit a foreign country, the vocabulary and expressions come to mind with greater facility. Priming, then, is quite different from the other types of memory in that it requires no conscious recollection but does reveal the effects of prior experience (i.e., memory). In contrast to episodic and semantic memory which involve "knowing when" or "knowing what," implicit memory has been characterized as "knowing how."

For an implicit memory task in the laboratory, an individual might be asked to engage in word puzzles, with no mention of a memory test. Try to complete the following fragments to form words: D_N_S_U_, AV_C_D_, T_QU_L_, A_R_V_R_, G_N_RA_I_N, and E_E_HA_T. Although it's fairly difficult, when the whole words have been seen previously, the number of fragments completed rises dramatically, providing evidence of memory.[1] This form of memory occurs even when individuals don't remember having seen the very same words! Even more striking, amnesics—who, by definition, have extremely poor episodic memory—perform at the same level as normals when an implicit test is used. For present purposes, this finding is of great interest because it shows that (1) it is possible to tap information stored in memory not normally available to consciousness, and (2) that separate memory systems can be differentially affected by factors such as aging and disease. We will see evidence that implicit memory is invulnerable to the effects of normal aging and may be spared in Alzheimer's disease as well.

MEMORY PROBLEMS: NORMAL AGING VERSUS ALZHEIMER'S DISEASE

Episodic Memory

The common stereotype that memory gets worse in old age actually is true for episodic memory but is not true for semantic memory or priming. Literally hundreds of laboratory studies have documented age differences in episodic memory tasks (e.g., memory for linguistic material such as words, sentences, paragraphs, and stories, and memory for visual material such as pictures, objects, faces, and scenes). Remember that these materials are presented for study and subsequently tested for retention by means of recall (e.g., write down all the words you can remember from that list) or recognition tests (e.g., shown a list of words, mark which ones you recognize). More recently, these age differences have been documented outside the laboratory as well (e.g., faces and names, hiding valuable objects, etc.).

These types of memory tasks are episodic because subjects are asked

---

1. The correct words for fragment completion are: *dinosaur, avocado, tequila, aardvark, generation,* and *elephant.* If you read this chapter from the beginning, the first three should have been easier than the last three.

to remember items experienced during a personally experienced episode. In a recent review of scientific studies (1993), I found that healthy older adults remembered an average of 32 percent less than young adults. This difference occurred even though memory was tested with picture recognition, probably the easiest episodic test (age differences are typically greater for free recall tests, in which no retrieval cues are provided). Thus, healthy elderly adults can be characterized—on a group basis—as having a measurable, *quantitative* loss of retrieval from episodic memory. (Robin West and her colleagues at the University of Florida have also found that age-related decline is the primary factor in "everyday memory performance.") The quantitative aspect is emphasized because the *manner* in which healthy older adults remember is not qualitatively different from younger adults.

In contrast, the episodic memory deficit in Alzheimer's disease patients is definitely *qualitative.* For starters, these patients certainly remember less information. In a number of studies, dementia patients consistently recalled considerably less information compared to healthy elderly of the same age. But even more importantly, the *way* in which Alzheimer's disease patients recall information is very different from healthy older adults. A couple of examples from my own research will illustrate this point. This research was conducted when I was at Duke University, in collaboration with Reed Hunt (University of North Carolina at Greensboro) and Frederick Schmitt (University of Kentucky).

In one study, we asked subjects to read a number of sentences. Some of the sentences were complete, such as "The gentleman opened the *door.*" Other sentences were incomplete and the subject was asked to supply the missing word, as in "The teacher taught the ————." Later, we provided each person with the subject of each sentence (e.g., *gentleman* and *teacher*) and asked them to recall the object (last word) of that sentence (e.g., *door* for the first sentence; class, student, etc., for the second sample sentence, depending on the word generated).

Even though older adults recalled less information, both young and older healthy adults' memory benefited from generating their own words. Words they thought of themselves (for incomplete sentences) were better remembered than words they read in the complete sentences. This phenomenon is known as the *generation effect.* The magnitude of this effect is plotted in figure 1 as the difference between generated minus read words. The Alzheimer patients, in contrast, did not benefit from the generation effect; they recalled words poorly regardless of whether those

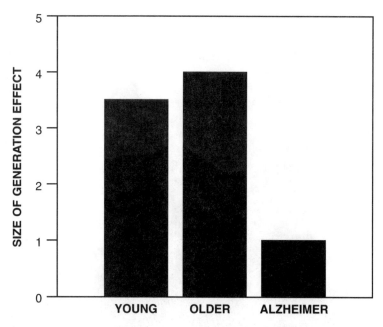

Fig. 1: Mean size of the generation effect (number of generated minus read words recalled) in young and older healthy adults and Alzheimer patients (adapted from Mitchell, Hunt, and Schmitt, 1986). Note that normal aging does not diminish the memory advantage of self-generated information, but that Alzheimer patients' memory demonstrates virtually no benefit from generation.

words had been read or thought up. Thus, their episodic memory functions in a qualitatively different way, since their memory performance was not sensitive to the generation effect.

Another episodic memory task we investigated was *reality monitoring,* which involves discriminating memory for internal thoughts from external perceptions or actions. For instance, as you drive to work one morning, you wonder if you actually turned off your electric coffee maker or only *thought* about unplugging it. Did you actually take your medicine or only think about taking it? We showed subjects all the complete and incomplete sentences they had seen earlier, with the incomplete sentences filled in with their own words. They were asked to decide which sentences were ones they had read, and which ones they had generated (completed). In figure 2, it is evident that healthy older adults were just slightly worse than young adults—a quantitative difference—but Alzheimer

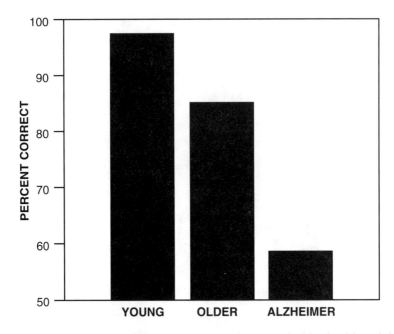

Fig. 2: Mean reality monitoring scores in young and older healthy adults and Alzheimer patients (adapted from Mitchell, Hunt, and Schmitt, 1986). Note that the ability to discriminate previously generated words from previously read words is only slightly impaired with normal aging, whereas Alzheimer patients have lost this ability.

patients performed much worse than either of the other groups. In fact, the Alzheimer patients' performance was no different from chance (50 percent), which is qualitatively different from the healthy older adults. This result parallels anecdotes about Alzheimer victims who have written the same check a few times, or who have left the range on.

Retrieval from Semantic Memory

When we speak, listen, read, or write; when we give someone directions to a favorite restaurant; or, when we think about a friend, we are retrieving information from semantic memory. The distinction between episodic and semantic memory was proposed by Endel Tulving in 1972; since then close to a hundred studies have focused specifically on semantic memory in the context of aging or dementia. The findings are quite clear: Normal aging does not impair semantic memory, while Alzheimer patients' ability to retrieve (remember) this kind of information deteriorates steadily over the course of the disease.

Retrieval from semantic memory can be tested in a number of ways. At the most basic level, people are simply asked what day it is, where they are, how to spell a word, and the like. Some studies have examined retrieval of general knowledge, such as historical or current events, vocabulary, names of famous people, and geography (e.g, what is the capital of Israel?). Laboratory studies typically employ tasks that yield easily quantifiable results, such as naming items from specified categories (e.g., list all the fruits you can think of, list as many U.S. presidents as you can), or simply naming specific objects or pictures (e.g., a key, a picture of an airplane).

Healthy older adults, as a group, rarely do worse than young adults on the foregoing kinds of tasks. In fact, a number of recent studies have found that older adults often perform significantly better than young adults on semantic memory tasks. For instance, in one study we conducted at Southern Methodist University (with Alan Brown, Todd Jones, and Laura Steen-Patterson) with current students (average age = 19) and older alumni (average age = 74), the older group's vocabulary scores were nearly 20 percent above those of the young. Other studies have found that memory for facts and world knowledge (e.g., history, entertainment, politics) also tends to actually *increase* with age.

In contrast, Alzheimer patients typically experience difficulty retrieving information from semantic memory. Early on, patients simply have problems retrieving specific names, a common memory complaint among healthy individuals as well. Frederick Schmitt and I found that relatively mild Alzheimer patients had more tip-of-the-tongues than age-matched healthy adults (e.g., shown a picture of an artichoke, the patients knew what it was, but couldn't retrieve the name). Another study by Jacob Huff and his colleagues at Massachusetts Institute of Technology also found naming impairments in Alzheimer patients. However, when given a name recognition test, as in "Is this called an *x*?" where *x* was the name of the accompanying line drawing, these patients performed as well as healthy control subjects. This suggests that the Alzheimer patients have not lost their semantic memory; rather, their *access* to information in semantic memory is impaired. There is further evidence of an access problem. Herbert Weingartner and his colleagues reported that more than two years before the onset of Alzheimer's, individuals in the Baltimore Longitudinal Study of Aging exhibited difficulty generating less common instances from certain categories such as fruits and vegetables. Even reading reflects this phenomenon. Karolyn Patterson and colleagues at the MRC Applied Psychology Unit in Cambridge, England, found impaired pronunciation of words with atypical spelling-sound correspondence (e.g., *busy* and *sew* were pronounced as "buzzy" and "sue").

A number of studies have analyzed the nature of the naming impairment in Alzheimer's disease. For some time, it was thought that the problem was primarily *perceptual*; in other words, the Alzheimer patients could not accurately interpret what an object was, which in turn prevented them from retrieving the correct name. For example, Howard Kirshner and his colleagues at Vanderbilt University found that Alzheimer patients made more naming errors for photographs of objects than for the actual objects. On the other hand, the healthy control adults actually made more perceptual errors than the Alzheimer patients did!

One problem is that many naming errors are not exclusively perceptual or semantic. For example, when a picture of a *pen* is called a "pencil" or a *chisel* is called an "ice pick," these names share both perceptual (long, thin, sticklike cylinders) and semantic (writing instruments, tools) attributes. Perceptual errors that have no apparent semantic component are actually quite rare (such as "bucket" for *thimble,* "wheel" for *button*). Likewise, semantic errors that have no visual or perceptual component (such as "saxophone" for a picture of a *harp*) are rare as well. However, pure semantic errors that are very common involve producing category superordinate names: "worm" for *caterpillar,* "vegetable" for *asparagus,* "bird" for *penguin,* and "bug" for *grasshopper.* Similarly, semantic errors recalling the *function,* but not the name, of the object are very common. For example, when asked to name pictured objects, an Alzheimer patient said that *sock* was "for a foot," *gun* was "pull trigger, say bam with that," and *ashtray* was a "cigarette dish." These functional errors tend to be more prominent and occur more often beyond the mild stages of the disease.

In light of the foregoing distinctions, studies by Kathryn Bayles and Cheryl Tomoeda at the University of Arizona and by myself and Frederick Schmitt have led to the conclusion that the source of the naming errors is *semantic* rather than perceptual. In other words, Alzheimer patients (at least in the mild to moderate range) *can* perceive objects, but have trouble accessing the specific name. Some investigators have interpreted the impaired access to semantic memory as involving *effortful* memory processes. In the next section, we will see evidence that implicit memory seems to be spared in the course of both normal aging and Alzheimer's disease.

Implicit Memory: An Invulnerable System?

As mentioned earlier, implicit memory appears to be the most basic memory system, and recent evidence suggests that it continues to function normally in old age, in amnesics, and perhaps in patients with Alzheimer's disease. Remember that some stimulus must be presented to the subject in order to elicit a response. Either the accuracy of the response (e.g., a subject completes a word fragment) or the speed of the response (e.g., a previously seen item is named faster) reveals the functioning of implicit memory.

An implicit memory task that I have used involves measuring how long it takes people to name pictures of common objects, such as line drawings of a dog, trumpet, banana, or a chest of drawers, etc. Naming time is measured in milliseconds from the moment a picture comes up on a computer monitor until an individual speaks into a microphone. Only naming times for names successfully retrieved are used in the analysis. When people are asked to name pictures a second time, their naming times are faster than on the first presentation indicating implicit memory for those pictures. This is true even for pictures that people cannot consciously recollect.

Frederick Schmitt and I employed this task with three groups of subjects: young and old healthy adults and Alzheimer patients. We asked them to name sixty pictures; half of the pictures were presented a second time a few minutes later. Average naming times (not shown) were fastest in young adults, somewhat slower in healthy older adults, and slowest in Alzheimer patients. In spite of the group differences in overall naming speed, the three groups showed equivalent increases in name retrieval speed on the second occurrence (or repetition) of a picture. The results for repeated picture naming are presented in figure 3. This phenomenon is called *priming* and is assumed to reflect the operation of implicit memory. Thus, neither normal aging nor Alzheimer's disease seems to disrupt the functioning of implicit memory. However, many researchers are actively investigating a variety of priming tasks, because while most of these tasks reveal preserved functioning in patients with Alzheimer's disease, some do not.

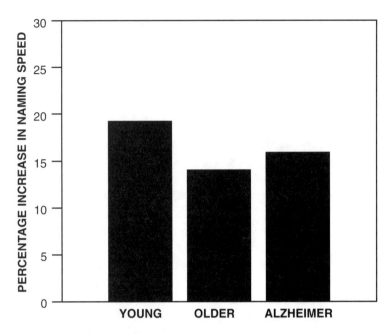

Fig. 3. Mean percentage increase in repeated picture-naming speed in young and older healthy adults and Alzheimer patients (from Mitchell and Schmitt). Note that all three groups benefit similarly from prior exposures to pictures.

A related finding has been reported by Laura Monti and John Gabrieli and colleagues at the Rush Alzheimer's Disease Center in Chicago. These investigators asked patients to read passages many times. Their Alzheimer patients showed normal implicit memory as evidenced by increased reading speed for identical passages on subsequent tests. This priming effect was equivalent for a group of normal elderly and the Alzheimer patients, in spite of the latter group's very poor performance on episodic (recognition) memory tests for the same passages.

Jason Brandt and his colleagues at Johns Hopkins University have employed another priming memory task. In this task, subjects are initially shown a list of words. Later, subjects see a longer list of words, some of which are related to the original list. Subjects are asked simply to say the first word that comes to mind—thus, it is not presented as a memory task. Both Alzheimer patients and normal elderly (mostly patients' spouses) revealed memory for the original words, in that their word associates to the new list tended to be the original words, at a greater-than-chance level. This priming memory equivalence held in spite of the Alzheimer patients' poor episodic recall (about 37 percent of the level of healthy older adults).

Daniel Schacter, at Harvard University, published a very interesting example of intact implicit memory in a patient (M.T.) diagnosed with Alzheimer's disease. Schacter took M.T. (an experienced "duffer" in his own words) out for a couple of rounds of golf. M.T.'s memory for the location of his last shot—episodic memory—was quite poor (only 35 percent correct). Likewise, his episodic memory for playing golf with Schacter was severely impaired, as he denied having played at all when asked about it a week after the fact. In contrast, his playing ability, and knowledge of etiquette, rules, strategies, and jargon demonstrated remarkable preservation of his semantic and priming memories. In light of the research discussed above, M.T.'s priming memory is not surprising. His semantic memory functioning, however, is unusually good compared to the average Alzheimer patient, but is in line with his laboratory measures, which show his vocabulary and information skills to be intact. His semantic memory functioning suggests that he is only in the mild stage at this point. It would not be surprising if his golf skills (i.e., priming memory) remain intact for some time after his naming and vocabulary abilities deteriorate in the course of the disease.

MEMORY TESTS AS DIAGNOSTIC CRITERIA

As we have seen, many episodic and semantic memory tasks distinguish dementia problems from minor memory problems associated with normal aging. Many of these kinds of items are part of existing diagnostic tests, such as the "Mini-Mental State" exam, developed by Marshal Folstein and others at Johns Hopkins University. Many researchers are working to develop language, memory, and other behavioral tests that more accurately discriminate Alzheimer's disease from other dementias. For example, Eileen Grist and Jane Maxim at Frenchay Hospital in England have developed the *Build-up Picture Test* for differentiating dementia from normal aging.

A reality monitoring test may be a useful addition to our current battery of assessment tools, as this test may tap memory problems that can lead to potentially life-threatening situations, such as forgetting to turn the stove off. Families with Alzheimer patients living at home should be attentive to situations that involve reality monitoring, such as locking doors, leaving appliances on, taking medications, and writing checks. Signs (e.g., *Is the stove off?* by the front door) and other external reminders (e.g., one box labeled for medicine not yet taken, another for medicine already taken) may be helpful.

Since many of the current medical tests are so expensive and are primarily useful only for exclusionary purposes, it behooves researchers to continue searching for simple behavioral tests that can help to positively identify dementia of the Alzheimer's type. Some of the priming memory tasks may prove to be useful for assessing what an individual's level of functioning was prior to the onset of the disease. Additionally, the *combination* of behavioral and the latest "high-tech" brain tests (e.g., PET, MRI, cerebral blood flow, and event-related potentials) may provide greater accuracy in diagnosis. Although there is no cure available at this time, early identification is a worthwhile endeavor, given its success in dealing with other diseases and the possibility of some kind of treatment.

TREATMENTS: NO CURE BUT SOME RELIEF

Three kinds of treatments are currently in practice: behavior management, drug therapy, and emotional support for the patient's caregiver. The last has been the most successful to date thanks to the untiring work of individuals (see chapter 12) and to the support provided by organizations such as the Alzheimer's Association. Behavior therapy holds no cures but it offers great improvement in the day-to-day management of patients with Alzheimer's disease and other dementia symptoms (see chapter 10). For instance, Veronique Breuil and her colleagues at Hopital Broca in Paris have reported some behavioral benefits following a "cognitive stimulation program."

Research on drugs that might enhance Alzheimer patients' performance on memory and language tasks is moving at a rapid pace. A computerized search restricted to a psychology database revealed 262 studies involving drugs and Alzheimer's disease just in the last ten years. A lot of work is being done with cholinesterase inhibitors (e.g., aminoacridines such as tacrine and velnacrine). These can prevent the rapid degrading of acetylcholine, an important neurotransmitter that Alzheimer patients typically have in reduced amounts. The logic is that a patient's limited supply of acetylcholine would have a better chance of doing its job if it can be kept from depleting so rapidly. There is also a lot of encouraging rescarch on the memory benefits of glucose, and some promising work on delayed onset of symptoms with anti-inflammatories. (For an update on drugs, see chapter 17 by Hutton and Hutton in this book.) With the number of new drugs being developed, the need is even stronger for better tests to positively identify Alzheimer's disease.

SUGGESTED READINGS

Bartlett, J. C., Halpern, A. R., and Dowling, W. J. "Recognition of Familiar and Unfamiliar Melodies in Normal Aging and Alzheimer's Disease." *Memory and Cognition* 23 (1995): 531–46.

Bayles, K. A., and Kazniak, A. W., with C. K. Tomoeda. *Communication and Cognition in Normal Aging and Dementia.* Boston: Little, Brown and Company, 1987.

Brown, A. S., and Rahhal, T. A. "Hiding Valuables: A Questionnaire Study of Mnemonically Risky Behavior." *Applied Cognitive Psychology* 8 (1994): 141–54.

Breuil, V., de Rotrou, J., Forette, F., and Tortrat, D. "Cognitive Stimulation of Patients with Dementia: Preliminary Results." *International Journal of Geriatric Psychiatry* 9 (1994): 211–17.

Davis, K. L., Thal, L. J., Gamzu, E. R., and Davis, C. S. "A Double-blind, Placebo-controlled Multicenter Study of Tacrine for Alzheimer's Disease." *New England Journal of Medicine* 327 (1992): 1253–59.

Edwards, J. A. *When Memory Fails: Helping the Alzheimer's and Dementia Patient.* New York: Plenum Press, 1994.

Folstein, M. F., Folstein, S. E., and McHugh, P. R. "Mini-Mental State: A Practical Method for Grading the Cognitive State of Patients for the Clinician." *Journal of Psychiatric Research* 12 (1975): 189–98.

Grist, E., and Maxim, J. "Confrontation Naming in the Elderly: The Build-up Picture Test as an Aid to Differentiating Normals from Subjects with Dementia." *European Journal of Disorders of Communication* 27 (1992): 197–207.

Huppert, F. A., Brayne, C., and O'Connor, D. W. *Dementia and Normal Aging.* Cambridge: Cambridge University Press, 1994.

Mitchell, D. B. "Semantic Processes in Implicit Memory: Aging with Meaning." In *Age Differences in Word and Language Processing,* edited by P. Allen and T. R. Bashore. Amsterdam: Elsevier Science, 1995.

Mitchell, D. B., Hunt, R. R., and Schmitt, F. A. "The Generation Effect and Reality Monitoring: Evidence from Dementia and Normal Aging." *Journal of Gerontology* 41 (1986): 79–84.

Monti, L. A., Gabrieli, J. D. E., Wilson, R. S., and Reminger, S. L. "Intact Text-specific Implicit Memory in Patients with Alzheimer's Disease." *Psychology and Aging* 9 (1994): 64–71.

Patterson, K. E., Graham, N., and Hodges, J. R. "Reading in Dementia of the Alzheimer Type: A Preserved Ability?" *Neuropsychology* 8 (1994): 395–412.

Pollen, D. A. *Hannah's Heirs.* New York: Oxford University Press, 1993.

Reisberg, B. (ed.). *Alzheimer's Disease: The Standard Reference.* New York: The Free Press, 1983.

Schacter, D. L. "Amnesia Observed: Remembering and Forgetting in a Natural Environment." *Journal of Abnormal Psychology* 92 (1983): 236–42.

Schneider, L. S. "Clinical Pharmacology of Aminoacridines in Alzheimer's Disease." *Neurology* 43, no. 8 (1993): S64–S79.

Strock, M. *Alzheimer's Disease.* Washington, D.C.: NIMH, 1994.

Tulving, E. "Organization of Memory: Quo Vadis?" In *The Cognitive Neurosciences,* edited by M. S. Gazzaniga. Cambridge, Mass.: MIT Press, 1995.

Vitaliano, P. P., Russo, J., Breen, A. R., Vitiello, M. V., and Prinz, P. N. "Functional Decline in the Early Stages of Alzheimer's Disease." *Psychology and Aging* 1 (1986): 41–46.

Weingartner, H. J., Kawas, C., and Rawlings, R. "Changes in Semantic Memory in Early Stage Alzheimer's Disease Patients." *Gerontologist* 33 (1993): 637–43.

West, R. L., Crook, T. H., and Barron, K. L. "Everyday Memory Performance across the Life Span: Effects of Age and Noncognitive Individual Differences." *Psychology and Aging* 7 (1992): 72–82.

9

Techniques for Enhancing Memory, Orientation, and Communication in the Alzheimer Patient

Doreen Kotik-Harper and Robert G. Harper

In the following essay, Doreen Kotik-Harper and Robert G. Harper, both clinical psychologists, give important practical information on how to facilitate communication with Alzheimer's patients, and how to keep these individuals actively involved with their environment. Even knowing what month it is becomes extremely difficult for those afflicted with Alzheimer's disease. All of us rely on cues in our environment to orient ourselves to place and time: we have calendars on the wall, wear watches on our wrists, and even use Christmas decorations to remind us that a special day will soon arrive.

To illustrate the importance of environmental cues to orient us to time, we offer the story of a woman with Alzheimer's disease who found Easter basket grass laying on the floor. The grass reminded her that holiday festivities were drawing near. She took the artificial grass to the dining table, which had large Easter lilies upon it. Her family fondly remembers her asking, "Would you like to put this on the tree?" She had apparently confused her favorite holidays. Perhaps her orientation to time was lost in this case, but her love of a good holiday was very much intact!

BASIC CONSIDERATIONS

Family members often ask if keeping the Alzheimer patient active, involved, and stimulated can stop the progression of the disease. While such intervention cannot "cure" or halt the dementing process, patients who are kept active and encouraged to take responsibility for themselves may experience a greater sense of physical well-being, self-control, and involvement in the family. It is clear that people with Alzheimer's disease cannot learn as well as before, because of the damage that has occurred to their brains. However, Alzheimer patients may be able to learn simple tasks and facts if they are repeated often enough. For example, demented persons who feel lost and confused in a new place can eventually "learn" to find their way around.

What is important is that family members keep their expectations of the patient reasonable and accept that certain skills may be lost forever. Pressuring the patient to learn, or providing too much stimulation and activity, can result in an inappropriately intense negative emotional reaction and cause guilt and anxiety.

Individuals who do not have brain impairment are able to focus their attention on the most relevant information in their environment, ignoring what is unimportant. We are able to scan a room quickly to see who is in the room and what is happening. We note pieces of furniture and knick-knacks, and we may be able to read a book and watch television at approximately the same time. Simultaneously, we take in information with our ears. We can listen to three kids, each asking for something different, be aware of the television show we are watching, and know that the baby is crying in the back room. All of this information can be taken in by focusing attention on what we are most interested in seeing, hearing, feeling, or tasting, and ignoring most of the other sources of stimulation.

For Alzheimer patients, who have difficulty focusing their attention, who forget even the most familiar of objects, and who have difficulty understanding speech and what is being asked of them, it is not surprising that going to a new place (or even familiar places) would be stressful and confusing. Imagine suddenly finding yourself in Hong Kong, where you know no one and cannot speak the language. Imagine how frightening that could be. What would you do in such a situation? Wander through the streets looking for something familiar? Perhaps find yourself asking the same questions over and over again? You might even become so frustrated that tears flow or you become angry.

What would help you feel more in control? Perhaps getting off the subway, going to a quiet park, getting away from all the strange sights and sounds would help reduce the anxiety and the restlessness. It would be reassuring if someone would communicate with you by slowly providing gestures, simple words, and maybe even pictures to help you understand where you are and what is happening.

Sometimes the most help we can provide the Alzheimer patient is finding ways to reduce unnecessary, unimportant stimulation, and providing very clear and focused information at an optimal level of intensity for the patient's level of functioning. At times the Alzheimer patient may withdraw from stimulation and actually become understimulated. The caregiver must become sensitive to providing appropriate levels of stimulation, drawing the patient in at times for active engagement, but being aware when the patient is becoming overaroused.

In the sections to come, we will attempt to show how to assess the patient's strengths and weaknesses so that caregivers may determine what levels and type of stimulation and communication are appropriate. Our goal is to work within the patient's range of capability, balancing stimulation, and breaking down (i.e., simplifying) activities so that the Alzheimer patient may continue to feel involved and somewhat in control of his or her destiny.

Diagnostic Issues

Although half of all dementias are caused by Alzheimer's disease, it is critical that other possible causes for impaired functioning in the elderly patient be evaluated and ruled out (see chapter 2) before caregivers and/or family members attempt to undertake enhancement programs. As the public becomes more aware of Alzheimer's disease, the danger of non-professionals making a diagnosis increases, and with it, well-intentioned but often inappropriate attempts or suggestions at management. If appropriate medical investigation is conducted, this should not be a problem, since a diagnosis of Alzheimer's disease in part depends upon a systematic exclusion of other dementing diseases, some of which are treatable or reversible.

Even where correct diagnosis is made, the caregiver should be alert to changes in the patient's thinking, speech, or emotions that may not be a true component of Alzheimer's disease. In some cases, such changes may reflect other, modifiable conditions, which, if taken into account, would reduce some of the confusion or disorganization that occurs in the demented patient. For example, demented individuals are vulnerable to delirium, which typically can be recognized as a sudden and obvious change in the patient's normal mental functioning. Delirium may have symptoms that are very similar to those of Alzheimer's disease, e.g., impaired alertness, slow and confused thinking, and difficulties in shifting or maintaining a focus of attention. However, these symptoms can result from various physical ailments or reactions to medicines (see chapter 2).

In addition, depression may or may not be present in the Alzheimer patient at a particular point in time. When present, depression can make impaired memory function even worse, reduce the patient's interest in the surrounding environment and in others, further compound difficulties in regulation of sleep, and even result in a full-scale withdrawal into a completely incapacitated vegetative state.

These considerations reflect that while Alzheimer's disease is progressive, the rate of progression and the way that the impairments show themselves may vary greatly across individuals and may be influenced by factors such as depression and toxic drug reactions. Though many strategies will be discussed here, it will be important to keep in mind that any management approach involves frequently changing interactions between the Alzheimer sufferer and the relative or caregiver. This is because the condition may vary from day to day and worsen over time.

WHAT IS COGNITIVE RETRAINING?

In recent years, a variety of techniques have been developed to help people with neurological diseases or brain injuries function more effectively. While these efforts have generated considerable excitement in the scientific community, this field of study is still in its infancy. It is still unclear just *how much* difference these approaches make and for *what kind* of brain impairment. For those with a family member who suffers from Alzheimer's disease, grief or desperation to help can tempt caregivers to *do everything* for their loved one. False hope should not be placed in some new development that has failed to stand the test of time and experience. Such an overreliance can be devastating to a family member who needs no additional undermining of morale.

Cognitive retraining is an approach that has been used with other kinds of brain-injured individuals who have experienced a blow to the head (often called a *closed head injury*) or a stroke. Presumably with both head injuries and stroke some areas of the cortex remain *intact*. Alzheimer's disease, however, is a degenerative disease that results in damage throughout the cortex of the brain, leaving no areas intact.

Many of the cognitive retraining approaches used with victims of stroke or head injuries involve working with some *internal* ability, that is, some aspect of brain functioning considered still to be intact. For example, a person with an injury to a language area of the brain may be trained to compensate for, or relearn, lost abilities by methods involving noninjured areas of the brain. Most techniques labeled *cognitive retraining* attempt to get the individual to use actively some ability to compensate or substitute for some deficit in reasoning, learning, or memory. We would caution against seeking help for an Alzheimer patient by enrolling in a program emphasizing *retraining*; this program ignores the fact that, at best, what one can hope to do is to delay an, as yet, unavoidable process of deterioration. Instead, *external* aids will be needed to compensate for the increasingly generalized deterioration.

In contrast, *reality orientation* approaches (which will be discussed in more detail later) emphasize use of *external* cues and structures to assist the Alzheimer patient in maintaining contact with the environment (e.g., calendars, written memory reminders). *Behavior modification* techniques (see chapter 10), in turn, emphasize the selective use of rewarding outcomes for desired patient behaviors (e.g., dressing independently, going to the bathroom without protest). Typically the rewarding events, or *reinforcers,* are praise, physical or social contact, or something the patient values. With appropriate external cues (e.g., praise), the Alzheimer patient may be expected to continue to act in the desired fashion as long as rewards occur with some frequency. It is especially important to realize, however, that behavior modification approaches with the Alzheimer patient depend upon the caregivers providing consistent use of reinforcers (rewards) when the desired behaviors occur.

MEMORY ENHANCEMENT

Aspects of Memory

Before we can attempt to "improve" memory functioning, we must first understand the different processes involved in forming memories. The ability to retain (remember) information from previous experience is one of our most important abilities on which our capacity to adapt and function effectively in different situations depends. Most people tend to think of memory as a single mental function, when in fact many mental processes are involved. First, we must *attend* (pay attention) to something before we can *acquire* (learn) information about it. Depending on the complexity of the information, some rehearsal (practice) may be required before it can be retained (remembered). Once acquired, this information is stored in what scientists have called *immediate* or *short-term* memory, where information we have just been exposed to is retained. Beyond this is a process of storage, where information in immediate memory is *consolidated* and finally retained in *remote* or *long-term* memory. When in the future we are exposed to familiar circumstances, we may *retrieve* (remember) certain information, such as the last meal ordered at a certain restaurant, or the like. Thus, memory involves attending, acquisition, and rehearsal (into long-term memory), and finally, retrieval. Disruption of any one aspect and memory will be impaired to some degree.

Experts often refer to a distinction between *semantic* and *episodic* memory (see chapter 8). Semantic memory involves information that is based on language, word knowledge, verbal concepts, and is independent of references to time or place. Episodic memory, in contrast, has to do with personally experienced events labeled in terms of time and place, such as a baseball game, a doctor's appointment, or a day at the office. Scientists who have studied memory in different age groups have noted that younger individuals rely more on episodic memory, whereas older persons use semantic memory more heavily.

It is also known that there are different brain centers for verbal, or language-based, information, and for nonverbal, or visuospatial information (forms, objects, geometric shapes, and directions). As we grow older our ability to deal with and recall nonverbal types of information declines, and with it our memory for shapes, forms, directions, and the like.

One can also distinguish between *recent* or *remote* memory. *Recent* memory refers to our ability to recall or recognize information or events within minutes, hours, or days, whereas events that occurred or information gained years ago are considered examples of remote memory. Unless some special area of the brain is damaged, our remote memories stay with us, even in the face of brain injury or neurological disease of the central nervous system. In contrast, our ability to retain recent information typically declines with age and with most diseases affecting the brain. In addition, depression can cause reversible impairments in recent memory.

Finally, whereas conscious memory for events and visual or language-based information (scientists call this *declarative memory*) declines with Alzheimer's disease, the ability to learn *how to do* things involving habits and simple routines, is preserved. An example of this *nonconscious procedural memory* would be dressing, doing physical therapy exercises, or grooming sequences. However, while an Alzheimer's patient could learn new motor behaviors of these kinds, he or she very well might not have any recollection of where or with whom the learning took place.

Memory Aids

Studies of the "normal" aging process suggest that, as we age, we may lose as much as 20 to 40 percent of our ability to deal with novel, unfamiliar situations and problems, spatial information, and recall of recent events. It also appears that older individuals stop using certain kinds of strategies for learning and recalling information that those with excellent or younger memories may use extensively. In recognition of this, psychologists specializing in the study of memory have developed some techniques for improving and enhancing memory functioning. Most of these techniques involve increasing the number of associations around the information we desire to retain. For example, making up a silly rhyme in connection with a certain word we need to remember may help us recall that word. The phrase *Every good boy does fine* helps us to remember the full notes E, G, B, D, F on the musical scale. Conjuring up an image that in turn is connected with some other kind of information (e.g., noting a resemblance between a certain person's face and features of a particular animal) may facilitate memory for that information. For caregivers it is crucial to keep in mind that Alzheimer's disease may keep the patient from generating helpful associations of either a verbal or nonverbal kind. In short, any memory improvement technique that depends upon new learning or novel experience should be regarded with caution, as the value of the approach will be quite limited.

In the case of Alzheimer's disease, memory is progressively impaired in a generally predictable order. Recent memory, especially for unfamiliar visuospatial information will be the first to deteriorate. Whereas the Alzheimer patient will seem to have a good memory for events that occurred in childhood or in earlier adulthood, he or she may get lost repeatedly, ask the same question, or never recall phone conversations or messages. As the condition worsens, gaps in remote memory may occur, even to the point that family members may not be recognized. Ultimately, even habits such as dressing and eating are disrupted and eventually lost.

Physical Aids

The order in which memory deteriorates, from the most unfamiliar and novel to the most repetitive experiences and behaviors, gives us a strategy for dealing with the Alzheimer patient. First, any enhancement technique that depends on new learning and recent memory is likely to fail, which may only frustrate and aggravate the problem. Where new things have to be learned, use of external aids, such as taking notes, will work best. For recall of time-related events, such as appointments, a calendar and even a digital alarm (some of which can be programmed to specify the information to be remembered), can help *substitute* for missing functions in the Alzheimer patient. (Be sure, however, that any electronic memory device is not so complicated that it is confusing or unusable.)

Association Aids

For the Alzheimer patient, making new bits of information part of old, well-known, and frequently repeated routine may help cue (elicit) recall of important new information. For example, having the patient take a new prescription at a time that had originally been set aside for administering a vitamin (for example, at breakfast), or when teeth are to be brushed (which places the patient in proximity to the medicine cabinet), would make it more likely that the medicine would be taken.

Backward Chaining

Learning new locations can be particularly difficult, or even beyond the capabilities of an Alzheimer sufferer, but a method called backward chaining has been helpful with some demented patients. Normally we learn to get from one place to another by learning various cues in a forward progression, from point of origin to destination. *Backward chaining* involves the opposite process, where the patient is taken first to the destination on repeated occasions, then familiarized with prominent locations increasingly distant from the destination and closer to the starting point. In a hospital setting, this initially might involve taking a patient from the bed, directly under supervision to the destination—say, the occupational therapy area. Subsequently, the patient would be taken to the closest landmark along the way, which might be the nurse's station, from which point the patient would try to get to the occupational therapy area.

This backward progression or "chaining" would be continued until the patient could walk from his or her room to various destination points with minimal or no supervision.

REMINISCENCE THERAPY

As the disease progresses, remote memory also begins to deteriorate. While nothing can stop this process, appropriate levels of stimulation and use of existing capabilities can be helpful. *Reminiscence therapy* or *reminiscence training* refers to an approach wherein the demented patient reviews past memories, in turn, using other mental functions that are exercised in a fashion that helps to maintain them. Scrapbooks of old photos with captions are often helpful as external aids in building a sense of history and meaningfulness in an individual who may be experiencing a sense of falling apart and futility.

While some or all of the techniques discussed above have been helpful to some demented individuals, none of them should be employed in hope of avoiding the requirement for frequent if not continuous supervision of the Alzheimer patient. At the very best, they might help compensate for the unavoidable but often unpredictable course of deterioration; at the least, appropriate use of these approaches can help organize the experience of the patient and structure the interaction between patient and family member in a way that enhances the quality of life for the Alzheimer patient.

Orientation

As mental functioning declines in the demented individual, the first things to be forgotten are the awareness of time, place, and self-recognition, in that order. The practical significance of such awareness or orientation is obvious: The level of independence and self-sufficiency an individual experiences depends upon this very basic ability to use information in the environment so that self, spatial location, and time of day can be identified. As the ability to recognize this information becomes less reliable, an individual loses control of many aspects of his or her life (e.g., getting around safely, self-medication, proper nutrition).

Determining an individual's level of orientation is relatively simple. Disorientation is generally judged to be present when an individual consistently (i.e., repeatedly over time) fails to respond correctly to questions pertaining to: one's own name and the names of familiar others; the place (including buildings, cities, and states); home address and telephone number; the time of day; and the date. Tests of orientation may also include other inquiries, such as date of birth, age, what the weather and season are, or the name of the current president. In assessing an individual's level of orientation, it is also very important to determine if reversible sensory impairment (i.e., hearing loss, diminished visual acuity) is contributing to the patient's confusion.

Reality Orientation

As disorientation about surroundings and the passage of time increases, confusion, frustration, or anxiety may cause withdrawal from others and result in less interaction with the environment and avoidance of excessive stimulation. Withdrawing from the world in this fashion, however, may cause an individual to be understimulated and *sensory deprived.* For the Alzheimer patient, whose thinking processes are already slowed and impaired, this lack of stimulation can cause even more confusion. To prevent understimulation in the demented individual, and to reestablish orienting behavior, a treatment approach called *reality orientation* was developed.

Reality orientation is based upon the belief that continual, repetitive reminders (information told to or shown to the demented patient by family members or caregivers, including the use of artificial props) will keep the patient stimulated and lead to an increase in orientation. The treatment of reality orientation usually involves two approaches. First, should the demented patient be in an institution, hospital, or day care setting, structured classes may be held several times a week, during which patients are asked to name common objects, identify colors, and perform other simple tasks. Second, and more importantly, the entire family or staff is trained to reorient and stimulate the patient's awareness during the entire day. This involves reinforcing (i.e., rewarding/acknowledging) the patient's accurate orienting statements and correcting the patient's inaccurate, confused statements.

The usefulness of reality orientation for the disoriented elderly has been the subject of much research. Although the findings have been mixed, in general, the approach is viewed positively by health care providers who work with confused older people. While the orienting benefits of this approach may not generalize much beyond the training setting (e.g., the hospital unit) individuals who receive reality orientation may interact more with others and their surroundings, and feel better about themselves. The increased sense of independence and control that this approach may engender in a confused elderly patient also results in the family member or caregivers feeling less burdened and more positive toward the patient.

The application of this approach is not limited to Alzheimer patients. It may also be of some benefit to elderly individuals whose confusion results from multiple strokes, medication effects, metabolic imbalances, nutritional deficiencies, sensory deprivation, dehydration, or emotional stress. It is important, however, that the well-meaning family member recognize when reality orientation may not be helpful. Cases where the approach probably should not be used would be when: (1) the dementing illness is rapidly progressive and considered to be terminal (e.g., certain brain tumors or cancer), (2) the demented patient has been totally disoriented or socially withdrawn for more than two years, and (3) the confused person reacts with intense anxiety or panic when encouraged to become oriented to present cues. In the last two cases, forcing patients to become more aware and oriented can result in more emotional harm and behavioral problems than letting them live in their own world. Retreat into self may be the only manner in which certain patients can tolerate their failing capabilities.

In order for reality orientation to be effective, reorienting techniques must be applied consistently by all people who come into contact with the patient, twenty-four hours a day. This requirement is more difficult than it sounds, as constant repetition and drilling of simple information with the confused individual can become boring and frustrating. It is up to the caregiver to make the reality training task a creative and challenging one. Reorienting the confused patient can occur informally throughout the day.

Some general guidelines do need to be kept in mind. Foremost among them is this: Treat the confused person with respect and dignity at all times. The demented family member should be addressed as though you expect him or her to understand. Recognize the individual's level of capability, but remember that you are dealing with an adult who should not be talked down to or treated as a child. Attempt to mention names of familiar people and objects, as well as the current date, the week, and the time of day in all conversations with the confused family member. Encourage attempts at personal care; doing the basic activities of daily living keeps the confused person in touch with reality. Reward the Alzheimer patient's attempts to increase awareness, and correct personal comments or those about the surroundings with a smile or a compliment. Do not accept confused, rambling, or mistaken beliefs about persons, places, or the time. With tact and support, correct the confused individual and return him or her to reality.

Materials Used to Enhance Orientation

Materials for encouraging reorientation and relearning are easy to find and need not be expensive. Of basic importance is the structuring of the patient's primary living space (e.g., the bedroom or the sitting room). Furniture and accessories should be kept neat and tidy, and in the same basic order. Ideally, the room should have a window, whereby the patient can tell the time of day and the weather. A large clock (preferably with a lighted dial) and a calendar should be visible. The patient should be encouraged to wear and use a watch that contains a date feature. Stimulating materials should be readily available for the patient, such as current newspapers, magazines, a radio, and a television. A daily schedule of the patient's hourly activities should be posted. Familiar accessories should surround the patient (e.g., family photos, mementos, favorite pieces of furniture, knick-knacks, and the like), and around major holidays the room may be decorated. To help keep the patient oriented to place, signs, directional arrows, night lights, or color-coding of doors may be helpful.

In addition to the ongoing orienting that should occur in every interaction with the patient, the family member may wish to have more structured periods of reality training. These times should be kept relaxed and informal so that they prove to be pleasant experiences for both you and the patient. These sessions should occur in the same setting, be kept short (about 10–15 minutes), and occur several times a week.

A standard prop employed in reality orientation classes is the reality orientation board. The type of board used can be cork bulletin board, pegboard, a felt board, a blackboard, or any surface that allows for an easy changing of information on a daily basis. A typical format for the reality board is:

Address is:
Today is:
The date is:
The year is:

The weather today is:
The next holiday is:
The next meal is:

The family member and the patient fill in the current responses to these sentence stems together. It is imperative that the reality board be kept current and correct. Other reality materials can include: a toy clock with moveable hands; photo albums and scrapbooks; flash cards with words and pictures; large-print books; magnetic alphabet boards; scrabble sets with large letters; county, state, and world maps; well-known landmarks or a United States map; a globe; large-piece jigsaw puzzle of animals, food, and common objects; plastic fruit and food; and large-print, illustrated dictionaries.

As noted throughout this chapter, the family member must remember that every Alzheimer patient has different strengths and weaknesses that change over time, and even vary somewhat from day to day. As such, it is up to the family member to decide which orienting and training techniques will be more suitable. For higher functioning patients in the early stages of the disease, discussion of current events and newspaper headlines, working on a simple crossword puzzle, or fill-in-the-blank statements may be appropriate. A moderately affected Alzheimer patient may be able to discuss such topics as recipes, television shows, short stories, or sports, and still be able to participate in simple card games or checkers. With the very demented and confused patient, the family member may do best to focus on constant repetition of personal information, such as name, address, telephone number, and the name of the important person in the patient's life (e.g., spouse, family member, or guardian). Such personal information should be typed on a permanent card that the patient carries at all times. The very confused and demented patient may also derive some benefit from the review of colors, names of objects, and the use of eating utensils or grooming objects.

In some cases the patient will be able to progress to somewhat higher levels of materials. Just remember not to set your expectations too high, and avoid abstract discussion or materials that can confuse and frustrate the patient. On the other hand, the patient should be stimulated and not bored. The key to reality orientation is that repetition and reminders should be offered in a positive, noncritical, and nonthreatening way. One of the primary goals of this technique is to rebuild the patient's self-confidence and restore personal dignity.

COMMUNICATIONS

As Alzheimer's disease progresses, language problems become more evident. The patient may ramble on, almost incessantly, in what may appear to be irrelevant, disorganized, repetitious, and fragmented sentences. In more advanced cases the patient may mumble unintelligible phrases or remember only a few key words (e.g., *yes* or *no*) which may be used inappropriately. Eventually the patient may be unable to speak at all. For most families, the patient's loss of effective speech is the most upsetting of all the Alzheimer symptoms. While confusion and memory loss may frustrate the family, the demented individual may still be perceived as the "same person." It is when Alzheimer patients have lost the ability to speak that families experience their loved ones as different from the persons they once knew. The family may believe that thoughts and feelings can no longer be shared with the patient; this may lead to fears that the patient experiences suffering without being able to communicate it.

Family members who are concerned about such issues must remember two important points. First, the severity of the patient's language impairment may not be an accurate indication of the degree of dementia. As previously noted, the symptoms and presentation of Alzheimer's disease may take many forms. In some patients, deficits in language may occur early in the illness; yet for other patients, language may remain relatively intact, while attention span, memory, or visual-spatial reasoning and coordination may be impaired.

Patients who have trouble vocalizing and producing logical speech may give the false impression that they are stupid or very impaired. Conversely, one might erroneously assume that if persons can repeat spoken instructions or read a set of directions, they should be able to carry them out. Not infrequently, such patients are judged to be cantankerous for not following directions (e.g., to eat or take medication at a certain time), when in fact they have severe problems in comprehending or executing directions. The second point to keep in mind is that spoken words are only part of a communication process. Patients with Alzheimer's disease may communicate their needs and feelings through nonverbal means (i.e., facial expression, body posture, and actions).

Families concerned about communication problems in the Alzheimer patient should first have auditory (hearing) and visual (seeing) perception and acuity tests performed, providing corrective devices (i.e, hearing aids or glasses) when appropriate. Families may also opt to have a speech therapist evaluate the Alzheimer patient who exhibits language problems. Such an assessment can help the family understand the type of speech disturbance the patient is experiencing, and also provide them with tips on how best to communicate with their loved one. The following are some general considerations to keep in mind when communicating with the Alzheimer patient who has language problems.

Communication Aids for the Alzheimer Patient
Who Has Problems Understanding Others

As discussed earlier, the Alzheimer patient has difficulty in correctly understanding what is going on in the surrounding world. First, older people in general have many more problems with their vision and hearing, which can cause confusion and uncertainty. Alzheimer patients have an added difficulty: they must make sense of (i.e., identify, organize, and process) the information that does reach their senses. This obstacle is compounded by difficulties pertaining to attention span, concentration, and memory. As noted earlier, a demented person may be able to repeat verbal instructions or read written directions without necessarily understanding, remembering, or being able to act upon them. Similarly, the patient may be able to understand a statement when delivered face-to-face, but fail to comprehend what is said over the telephone. The following suggestions should be helpful in communicating messages to the Alzheimer patient.

1. Make certain the patient hears you by speaking loudly (but not so loud as to frighten), standing face-to-face, and maintaining eye contact.

2. If you do need to raise your voice to be heard, lower the tone (pitch). A high-pitched voice may suggest to the patient that you are upset. The tone of your voice should always reflect calmness, reassurance, and the sense that you are in control of the situation.

3. Use overemphasis and exaggerated facial expressions to stress your point. Hand gestures and pointing to objects can be very beneficial in conveying a message.

4. Distracting or competing noises and activities should be eliminated. Alzheimer patients experience tremendous difficulty sorting out stimuli and focusing their attention.

5. Use short words and simple sentences (no more than four words) conveying only one message or thought.

6. Begin each sentence by addressing the patient by name and by identifying yourself if necessary. Use only nouns; avoid the use of pronouns (e.g., it, she, they).

7. Ask only one simple question at a time. Do not include complex or multiple choices in a question (e.g., "Do you want to visit John or Cousin Sue, or wait and go shopping later?"). If you must repeat a question, attempt to repeat your words exactly.

8. Break each task into simple steps and ask the person to do one step at a time. Most of the things that we ask the patient to do (e.g., get dressed, take a bath, brush teeth) are actually composed of a number of sequential tasks. The Alzheimer patient may not be able to sequence the events.

9. Speak slowly and wait for the person to respond. What seems like a long and unproductive silence to you may reflect the Alzheimer patient's attempts to concentrate, comprehend, and formulate a response. If the response does not come in one or two minutes, repeat your question exactly.

10. Use humor in your communication whenever appropriate and encourage the patient to express humor, especially in difficult and trying situations.

11. Even with patients who have severe language problems, do not assume that the patient *never* understands you. Abilities fluctuate and it is inconsiderate and demeaning to talk in front of the patient as though he or she were not there.

Communication Aids for Patients
Who Have Trouble Expressing Themselves

Alzheimer patients frequently have considerable difficulty expressing themselves, which can lead to feelings of frustration in both the patient and the family. Such problems in communication may precipitate an emotional outburst in the patient (e.g., bursting into tears or storming out in a fit of anger), because it is felt that no one understands. How you attempt to help the demented person's self-expression will depend upon the type of difficulties the patient experiences as well as his or her personality and temperament.

For instance, some patients who suffer from *anomia,* or difficulty in naming things, may become quite annoyed and even angry if a caregiver intervenes to provide the correct word. Such patients may find it hard to accept their disabilities and their increasing dependence upon others. Some patients may feel less frustrated and be appreciative if they are supplied with the correct word rather than left on their own to search and struggle for it. If the patient has used the wrong word and you are not certain what is being talked about, you may ask that the object be pointed out and described.

At other times, the only way to determine what a patient is trying to communicate is to make a series of guesses. In some cases this may require taking into consideration not only the words the patient has provided, but also the manner in which they are presented (e.g., anxiously concerned, assertive and demanding, nervous and restless). For example, a patient may constantly make some inquiry about food. Efforts to explain when the next meal might arrive or describing the menu seem not to alleviate the concern. Such a patient may be expressing fears of being cared for properly and the need for reassurance.

For patients who can say only a few words, or shake and nod their heads, it is necessary to set up a regular routine and a standard set of questions for checking on their well-being. If these patients appear to be in distress, go through a checklist of what might be ailing them, proceeding slowly and checking on one point at a time (e.g., Are you hungry? Are you cold? Do you need to use the bathroom?). Point to body parts rather than naming them (e.g., Does this hurt?). The key points to remember are: convey your patience and concern to the demented person, and check each of your guesses with the patient to determine their correctness.

Nonverbal Communication

Much of this section has made reference to the manner in which the caregiver and the patient may communicate without the use of spoken language (i.e., through posture, gestures, and facial expressions). This type of communication actually goes on all the time even when speech is used (e.g., avoiding eye contact when ashamed, tensing body posture when angry, tapping the hand or foot in impatience). It is extremely important for the family member to read or interpret what the patient's behavior is conveying, and to also be aware of the nonverbal messages that are sent to the patient.

In communicating with the Alzheimer patient, first determine if the patient is *receptive* and listening to what is being said. The receptive, attentive patient will appear relaxed in facial expression and in muscle tone, will extend a hand or offer verbal greeting, will smile and nod to statements, will sit or stand still, will maintain eye contact, will lean forward or cock the head to one side to hear better. A *nonreceptive* listening patient turns away from the speaker, avoids direct eye contact, does not nod in affirmation or ask questions for clarification, may appear confused, appears restless or walks away, frowns, has general body muscle tension, fidgets or shakes, may appear anxious, or pulls away from physical contact. If the patient appears to be nonreceptive because of some negative emotional state (e.g., fear, panic, or anger), it may be best to leave him or her alone rather than risk escalating feelings. You may want to let the patient know that you realize he or she does not want to talk now and that you will return later. Never try to force a patient to do something.

The following are some suggestions on how to increase your ability to express yourself with the nonverbal patient.

1. Caring for the Alzheimer's patient can generate chronic feelings of fatigue and frustration. You must be careful, however, not to convey these feelings through body language, as they may upset or agitate the patient. Strive to maintain a calm exterior and remain pleasant and supportive.

2. Even a severely demented and noncommunicative patient needs affection. Smile, hold the patient's hand, place your arm around the person, or provide an occasional hug.

3. Touching can also be a more direct and effective technique for communication, e.g., redirecting the patient back to the task at hand, inhibiting an undesirable response, or calming and reassuring the patient.

4. Look directly at the patient, and sense the person's receptiveness; if necessary hold off on your communication until later when he or she is more able to listen.

5. Use gestures, point, touch, and hand the patient objects. Use pantomime or direct action for purposes of demonstration and imitation (e.g., brushing the teeth).

Communication with an Agitated Patient

A final and important point concerns how to recognize growing agitation and negative emotion in a patient. Frustration, fear, hostility, and aggression in the Alzheimer patient may be communicated through general increase in body movement and agitation, such as restless, rapid pacing; kicking doors or rattling door knobs; pushing furniture about; making fists or waving arms; facial changes, such as grimacing, frowning, or darting eyes; changes in voice, such as an increased volume, speech, and tone; and physical changes, such as rapid breathing, widening of the eyes, dilating pupils, and tightening of muscle tone. When a patient demonstrates such signs of agitation, approach the person with calmness and reassurance; reduce the surrounding stimulation (e.g., turn off the television or radio, and have others move away); remove dangerous objects from the area; do not pressure the patient or make additional demands; and make certain that all your communications, both verbal and nonverbal language, are consistent. In such stressful situations, the patient's memory loss may work to your advantage. Distracting the patient or removing the individual from the situation may make it difficult for him or her to remember what was so upsetting.

WHOM TO CONSULT

A final question can be asked: Who is qualified to provide the services that have been described in this chapter—cognitive retraining, behavior modification, and reality orientation? While many different professionals may have had specific training in utilizing these techniques (this of course should be verified at the outset of any treatment, irrespective of any other credentials the provider may have), typically they are provided by certain disciplines. In particular, psychologists are trained in behavior modification techniques, as well as cognitive retraining approaches. Speech pathologists are trained to work with brain-injured patients, utilizing cognitive retraining methods. Many psychologists, speech pathologists, and occupational therapists use reality orientation techniques with demented and brain-injured patients. Irrespective of the type of professional, the quality of care is always important, and this issue can be best addressed through consultation with a trusted physician, or through contact with reputable agencies or organizations specifically devoted to helping Alzheimer patients and their families. The important thing to keep in mind is that, as yet, the best one can do is to fight disuse and to help the Alzheimer patient maximize personal functioning. Any approach that promises more than that should be regarded with suspicion and investigated carefully.

SUGGESTED READINGS

Albert, M. S., and Moss, M. G. "The Assessment of Memory Disorders in Patients with Alzheimer's Disease." In *Neuropsychology of Memory,* 2d ed., edited by L. R. Squire and N. Butters. New York: Guilford Press, 1993.

Bartol, M. A. "Nonverbal Communication in Patients with Alzheimer's Disease." *Journal of Gerontological Nursing* 5 (1979): 21.

Burnside, I. *Working with the Elderly: Groups Process and Techniques,* 2d ed. Monterey, Calif.: Wadsworth Health Sciences Division, 1984.

Drummond, L., Kirchhoff, L., and Scarborough, D. "A Practical Guide to Reality Orientation: A Treatment Approach for Confusion and Disorientation." *Gerontologist* 18 (1978): 568.

Harvard Mental Health Letter. *Alzheimer's Disease—Part 1.9,* no. 2 (1992): 1.

Harvard Mental Health Letter. *Alzheimer's Disease—Part 2.9,* no. 3 (1992): 1.

Hussian, R. A. *Geriatric Psychology: A Behavioral Perspective.* New York: Van Nostrand Reinhold, 1981.

Patterson, R. L., Dupree, L. W., Eberly, D. A., Jackson, G. M., O'Sullivan, M. J., Penner, L. A., and Kelly, C. D. *Overcoming Deficits of Aging: A Behavioral Approach.* New York: Plenum Press, 1982.

Poon, L. W., Fozard, J. L., Cermak, L. A., Arenberg, D., and Thompson, L. W., eds. *New Directions in Memory and Aging: Proceedings of the George A. Talland Memorial Conference.* Hillsdale, N.J.: Lawrence Erlbaum, 1980).

Taulbee, L. R., and Folsom, J. C. "Reality Orientation for Geriatric Patients." *Journal of Hospital and Community Psychiatry* 17 (1966): 23.

Yesavage, J. A. "Imagery Pretraining and Memory Training in the Elderly." *Gerontology* 29 (1983): 271.

Zarit, S. H., Cole, K. D., and Gruder, R. L. "Memory Training Strategies and Subjective Complaints of Memory in the Aged." *Gerontologist* 21 (1981): 158.

10

Behavioral Management of Secondary Symptoms of Dementia

Paul K. Chafetz

As Alzheimer's disease progresses, the affected individual frequently behaves in unusual ways, and these new behaviors may embarrass family members when carried out in public. Unfortunately, some caregivers feel so self-conscious that they further restrict their social activities. It may prove helpful if the caregiver can find humor in such situations, rather than suffer embarrassment.

A spouse related an incident concerning her Alzheimer husband that stirs fond memories. She and her husband were having a hamburger at a take-out restaurant when she noticed that her husband's pants were unzipped. When she pointed this out to him, he was completely undisturbed and saw no reason to correct this unimportant problem. As he explained to his wife, "Oh well, it's not going anywhere."

Some Alzheimer behaviors may develop that create problems for the patient or the caregiver. The unzipped pants were not perceived as a problem by the patient but they posed an awkward situation for his wife. According to Paul K. Chafetz, a clinical psychologist, many behaviors that create problems for the Alzheimer patient and the caregiver can be humanely altered by applying principles of behavior modification. His essay provides an overview of such behavioral management principles and some practical information that may serve as a useful guide to the caregiver in attempting to modify unwanted patient behaviors.

The *primary* and defining symptoms of dementia refer almost exclusively to declines in such *cognitive* abilities as intellect, memory, language, and executive function. *Secondary* symptoms of dementia, however, are those *behaviors* that disturb other people, place excessive demands on caregivers, disrupt the patient's environment, or threaten the patient's own well-being.

The distinction between primary and secondary symptoms of dementia is extremely important. This is because *primary* symptoms usually cannot be much improved with today's health care tools, while *secondary* symptoms, if properly recognized, can often be significantly improved with existing methods. In Alzheimer's disease, the progressive loss of mental abilities is directly linked to progressive damage of brain tissue caused by physical illness. Since many details of this disease process are still inadequately understood, little or nothing can currently be done to stop or reverse it.

Secondary symptoms, in contrast, are, in large measure, responses to the particular environment in which the patient functions. *Environment* refers to all sources of stimulation available to the patient, including people, animals, objects, colors, temperatures, smells, and so on. Even such factors as personality, personal history, and current life situation are believed to have a significant controlling influence on the behavior of demented individuals. Unlike the reality of unchangeable brain tissue disease, environmental conditions that have allowed undesirable behaviors to develop can be changed. It would be tragic and foolhardy not to pursue aggressively the therapeutic options that behaviorism presents.

THE BEHAVIORAL APPROACH

Overwhelming evidence exists that behavior modification techniques are effective in managing many secondary symptoms among institutionalized dementia victims. These techniques are designed to increase desired behaviors (e.g., going to the restroom to urinate) and to reduce undesirable behaviors (e.g., disrobing in public).

Behavioral techniques are grounded in a rehabilitative, behavioral-ecological model, which requires close examination of the interdependence of the patient and his particular environment. The basic premise of this perspective is that most behaviors are learned, including healthy, sick, and aged behaviors. This is referred to as *behavioral plasticity*. Because these behaviors are learned, they can be corrected and possibly prevented. This also suggests that decline is not universal. Not all demented individuals display the same disruptive behaviors, nor are all disruptive behaviors irreversible. Another major premise of this approach is that of *dynamic interdependence,* meaning that a behavior is in large measure determined by environmental variables.

Secondary symptoms that psychologists are often able to treat by behavior modification include *behavioral excesses* (behaviors that cause problems due to the increased incidence or increased intensity of normal behaviors); *behavioral deficiencies* (behaviors that do not occur in sufficient frequency or intensity); and *behaviors that are inappropriate in their timing, location, or target* (behaviors that *are* normal in other circumstances).

Behavioral excesses include complaints, requests, repetitive vocalizations or movements, elation, rapid talking, pressure of speech, screaming, verbal abuse, self-injurious behavior, physical aggression, belligerence, irritability, physical agitation, restlessness, anxiety, and fearfulness. *Behavioral deficiencies* include the reduction or lack of: socializing, participation in activities, talking, self-feeding, self-toileting, self-grooming, walking, and cooperating with caregivers. *Behaviors that are inappropriate in their timing, location, or target* include disrobing in public; eloping; inappropriate elimination; inappropriate sexual behavior; insomnia/hypersomnia; and trespassing to the wrong room, bed, or closet. Most behavior problems among nursing home residents tend to be problems of behavioral excesses. Behavioral deficits are also very common, while problems of inappropriate timing, location, or target (stimulus control) are less frequent.

BASIC BEHAVIORAL PARADIGMS

Virtually all behavioral methods for improving patient functioning derive from two traditional behavioral paradigms. The first is called the *classical* or *respondent* model of learning, and is most associated with Ivan Pavlov, a Russian psychologist active in the 1920s. This paradigm focuses on behaviors that are largely involuntary and controlled by the body's autonomic nervous system. Examples of such behaviors include salivation, heartrate, and emotional states.

The second behavioral paradigm is called the *operant* model, and is usually associated with B. F. Skinner, an American psychologist active from the late 1930s to the 1980s. This paradigm focuses on behaviors that are conscious, voluntary, and purposeful, and are controlled especially by the cerebral cortex. Speech and all observable motor behaviors (except reflexes and involuntary movements) would be included.

This model reasons that all voluntary behavior is influenced by its context. That is, through experience, individuals learn that observable environmental conditions make it possible to guess pretty accurately whether a particular behavior by the organism will bring to it a pleasant or unpleasant consequence. This idea is summarized as "SORC," which stands for

Stimulus (also called discriminative stimulus, antecedents, cues, or prompts)

Organism (the abilities and limitations created for an individual by its genetic, physiological, historical, and social characteristics)

Response (the behavior itself)

Consequence (also called reinforcement, reward, punishment, and the like).

Examples of such operant learning pervade our lives. We all recognize the discriminative stimulus of a phone ring. We respond by picking up the phone and saying hello because we have so often been reinforced for such behavior by hearing the caller's voice. Experiencing the sight, sounds, and smells (cues) of a ballgame in a ballpark elicits specific behaviors (like cheering) that may be considered strange in other contexts. Many common situations become cues for us to choose to act in specific ways, and then reward us for so acting.

Most instances of voluntary, inappropriate, learned behavior by dementia victims involve the patient responding to whatever *cue* is most noticeable and subjectively relevant at the moment. So, for example, seeing a door, especially a glass door or open door, will attract any patient who is restless and enjoys walking, or who feels lost and wants to *go home*. The door is a cue that elicits exiting behavior because, in previous experience, walking-through-door behavior has led to gratification in the form of strolling or getting home.

Learning becomes random when caregivers allow the *links* (also called *contingencies*) between desired patient behaviors and pleasant consequences to weaken or dissolve. If caregivers do not carefully insure that pleasant consequences follow most acceptable actions, random environmental events will establish haphazard, even dangerous, new *rules* for patients to live by.

For example, when the patient's dementia causes a decreased sense of social propriety, and caregivers do not provide the patient with structured activities, several behaviors are likely to emerge because they are available on the patient's own body, and because they feel good. Some are often unacceptable, such as skin scratching, nose-picking, anal digging, and masturbation. Others are sometimes acceptable, unless their frequency is very high, such as patting, rubbing, rocking, walking, and tapping. These *self-stimulatory* behaviors are self-reinforcing, and usually indicate inadequate environmental stimulation.

Much undesired patient behavior is inadvertently reinforced by caregiver attention. Speech—such as questions, statements, or moans—that is disruptively loud or repetitive almost always results in increased caregiver attention. Contrary to *common sense,* waiting longer to respond to the patient for such behavior may actually strengthen, rather than weaken, the behavior. This is because it *trains* the patient that extensive responding is simply required to gain the attention reward.

It is crucial to realize that these two behavioral paradigms, the classical and the operant, are useful in understanding the development of *both* appropriate, desirable behaviors, *and* inappropriate, undesirable, even self-destructive behaviors. By applying these concepts to the secondary symptoms shown by dementia victims, in what is called a *functional analysis of behavior,* it is possible to both understand the behavior better and design interventions that may improve the patient's behavior.

In dementia sufferers, learning is, by definition, very inefficient. Therefore, it is vital that caregivers continually enable, prompt, and reward appropriate behavior.

PRINCIPLES OF OPTIMAL BEHAVIOR MANAGEMENT

Most caregivers readily understand the importance of providing ongoing quality health care, nutrition, hygiene, and affection for their dementia patient. The following list of additional concepts will help caregivers minimize the burden presented by secondary symptoms in dementia.

1. Reward desired behaviors every time. This means simply a kiss, a touch, a smile, a *thank you.* To the greatest extent possible, ignore undesired or inappropriate behaviors. This means showing no emotion, not making eye contact, and not speaking of the undesired behavior.

2. Provide daily activities involving movement to music (dancing, marching, exercising, singing and swaying, etc.). A portable tape player and radio will prove very handy.

3. Foster any and all remaining skills that are appropriately independent. Let the patient help with tasks, however small, that he or she can still do. Avoid routinely doing things that the patient can do. Give no more help than is needed.

4. Choose some desired behaviors that are too infrequent, and work at increasing them. This is more likely to prove helpful than if you focus on decreasing some frequent, undesirable behaviors. Prompt, invite, and encourage the patient to participate in appropriate activities.

5. Simplify complex behavioral sequences into small segments. Eating a meal, for example, consists of sitting down at the table, picking up a fork, spearing the food, raising it to the mouth, and so forth.

6. Decide, based on your observation of the patient, what his optimal level of stimulation is, then try to provide it. Pay attention to lighting, noise, and the number of people around.

7. Foster routine by maintaining a consistent schedule and consistent way of doing things.

8. Whenever possible, avoid, delay, limit, minimize, and shorten the use of mechanical restraints, and (with physician approval) sedating medicines.

9. Provide multiple, redundant sensory cues. For example, to help the patient locate kitchen or bedroom items, cabinet doors and drawers may be labeled with pictures and names of the contents.

10. Modify the environment to improve the patient's access to appropriate places and materials, and to reduce his access to inappropriate places and materials. This will increase the probability of appropriate activities and behavior. Use locks or spring latches on doors, drawers, and cabinets to prevent dangerous access; use labels and pictures to encourage access.

11. Never assume that a behavioral or cognitive symptom is inevitable and irreversible. Always search first for a treatable cause of the symptom. Daily possibilities to watch for include pain, hunger, thirst, and drug side effects.

12. If you cannot figure out why a certain behavior problem continues, keep a behavioral logbook. Record, each hour, what happened before and after each episode of the behavior. This will help identify hidden links between cues, behaviors, and rewards.

13. If you still do not know how to master a particular situation, call the appropriate specialist. This may be a psychologist, psychiatrist or other physician, nurse, or social worker. To locate such specialists, contact the appropriate department of the nearest university, major hospital, or medical school. Also, psychological and other professional organizations may be located in the yellow pages.

14. Caregivers must take good care of themselves, too. They should assertively seek the support, reassurance, and assistance of friends and relatives. Caregivers should educate themselves about dementia through reading and attending Alzheimer support group meetings. They should fully use the skills of knowledgeable professionals who are available to them.

15. Avoid confrontation with the dementia sufferer over any factual issues. If he or she holds firmly to an inaccurate belief or dislikes some facts which can be grasped accurately, the caregiver should not be drawn into arguments. Instead, the caregiver should (a) be *non-committal* about the facts ("My goodness! I just don't know!" or "We'll have to check on that"), and (b) show *empathy* for the patient's feelings ("That must be awful! I hear you!").

ADDENDUM

Example 1

Mr. Scott (not his real name) is a seventy-year-old retired postman who lives at home with his wife. After three years of noticeable cognitive decline, he is now moderately demented. He gets good medical care, and is otherwise healthy. His wife has become knowledgeable about his condition, and she has family members who visit and assist her.

Mr. Scott has not been a major behavioral problem until recently. In the past month, he has had occasional angry outbursts. At these times, he stands up, paces, raises his voice to curse and shout commands or demands, grabs onto someone's arm too tightly, and sometimes raises his hand menacingly. Usually he ceases after Mrs. Scott starts to cry and begs him to stop. Mrs. Scott is afraid he will injure her or someone else, or provoke others to hit him. She worries more than before, and is becoming somewhat demoralized.

To understand this difficult situation, we must realize that such behavior is not a pure or inevitable result of progressive brain impairment. Rather, it results from certain *combinations* of (a) brain impairment and (b) environmental stimuli and consequences.

Because of his impaired brain function, Mr. Scott is much less able to make his needs known, to understand accurately social situations, to tell the difference between safe and dangerous situations, and to inhibit his emotional responses. In an ideal environment, these limitations would be no problem, because he would never encounter ambiguous situations or experience unpleasant emotions. In the real world, however, new or unfamiliar social situations are unavoidable, and no caregiver can anticipate a dementia victim's every need.

While dementia *predisposes* victims to certain unpleasant behaviors, it is often actually the response of caregivers that determines whether the behavior will appear. Angry outbursts often appear to "suddenly come out of nowhere," though, in fact, they usually take from minutes to hours to develop. Early, appropriate intervention by an attentive caregiver can often nip an emerging problem in the bud.

The key is to *develop a good sense of which of the victim's needs is going unmet at the moment.* Table 1 lists the most common need states.

Based on familiarity with the dementia sufferer, his habits, and his recent schedule, the caregiver can often make a good guess as to which need is being frustrated. Next, the caregiver takes steps to satisfy the unmet need. She should talk reassuringly, gently but firmly separating him from the current situation, and bringing him to wherever the unmet need can be quickly gratified. Surprise and returned anger should be avoided. Armed with this knowledge, Mrs. Scott began to realize that Mr. Scott's "sudden rages" usually occurred during or soon after a visit by a male relative, during which he was excluded from, and unable to understand much of, the conversation. He was therefore bored and lonely. Mr. Scott's impaired thinking allowed him to develop the self-esteem-protecting delusion that this interloper was having an affair with his wife.

Mrs. Scott decided to include her husband more in conversations with visitors. To assure herself the opportunity to have private conversations, she asked visitors to come in pairs. One visitor was therefore always

TABLE 1
NEEDS AND NEED STATES

Needed Commodity	*Need State*
Food	Hunger
Drink	Thirst
To Void	Bowel or Bladder Pressure
To Cool Off	Feeling Hot, Sweating
Warmth	Feeling Cold, Shivering
Looser Clothing	Discomfort at Openings
Exercise	Motor Restlessness
Affection, Socialization	Loneliness
Sleep	Fatigue
Quiet Time	Overstimulation, Agitation
Sensory Stimulation	Boredom
Reassurance	Fear, Anxiety
Empathy	Suspicion, Anger
Medical/ Nursing Evaluation & Treatment	Pain

available to chat with Mr. Scott. After each visit, Mrs. Scott took care to show affection to her husband. The result was that his outbursts became very infrequent, and Mrs. Scott's confidence returned.

Example 2

Mrs. Reynolds is a seventy-eight-year-old widow living alone in an apartment building for able-bodied elderly persons. Mild dementia has been present for one year. She is maintaining a good level of social interaction, but recently those around her have noticed her body odor and that she looks unwashed and unkempt. Yet Mrs. Reynolds's appetite, mood, orientation, and other behaviors are not deteriorating.

This is a relatively straightforward example of a behavioral deficit resulting from inadequate environmental input. The staff's optimal approach is to assume that Mrs. Reynolds (a) has *not* lost the *ability* to perform personal hygiene activities, but (b) has lost the ability, at least temporarily, to remember on her own to perform them. Intervention consists of building two elements into Mrs. Reynolds's day. First are stimuli that encourage washing, such as prompts, requests, reminders, opportunities, and offers of assistance. Second are positive consequences that reward her for washing, such as praise, compliments, affection, and words of appreciation or admiration.

Example 3

Mrs. Hawthorne is a seventy-year-old, mildly demented female nursing home resident. Though often observed walking around her room, she quickly sits down whenever staff enter her quarters, insists that she cannot walk, and demands to be transported in a wheelchair. When staff try to help her to stand or walk, she acts lame, like "dead weight." When the maintenance man came to fix her sink, she slid from the bed to the floor *three times,* each time pleading with him until he lifted her (again, like "dead weight") back onto her bed.

As was true with Mrs. Reynolds, an explicit program of prompting and rewarding the deficient but desired behavior (walking unassisted) is in order. It is often difficult, however, to find something that is rewarding to people like Mrs. Hawthorne. Though her behavior communicates great dependency, she often seems depressed and claims to have no interest in anything. In such cases, remember the Premeack principle (Rimm and Masters, 1979, pp. 171–73), which states that the privilege to engage in preferred activities may be used to reinforce less preferred behaviors. Mrs. Hawthorne very much enjoys her son's weekly visits. With his cooperation, the staff informed her that she could earn additional brief visits by him if she resumed walking to the table at mealtime. This plan was successful, and was extended to walking to activities, and so forth.

Suggested Readings

Baltes, M. M., and Barton, E. M. "New Approaches toward Aging: A Case for the Operant Model." *Educational Gerontology: An International Quarterly* 2 (1977): 383–405.

Haley, W. E. "Priorities for Behavioral Intervention with Nursing Home Residents: Nursing Staff's Perspective." *International Journal of Behavioral Geriatrics* 1 (1983): 47–52.

Hussian, R. A. "Geriatric Behavior Therapy." In *Geriatric Mental Health,* edited by J. P. Abrahams and V. Crooks. Orlando, Fla.: Grune and Stratton, 1984.

Hussian, R. A. and Davis, R. L. *Responsive Care: Behavioral Interventions with Elderly Persons.* Champaign, Ill.: Research Press, 1985.

Maletta, G. J., and Pirozzolo, F. J. "Assessment and Treatment of Behavioral Disturbances in the Geriatric Patient." In *Behavioral Assessment and Psychopharmacology,* edited by F. J. Pirozzolo and G. J. Maletta. New York: Praeger, 198 1.

Rimm, D. C., and Masters, J. C. *Behavior Therapy Techniques and Empirical Findings,* 2d ed. New York: Academic, 1979.

Rosberger, Z., and MacLean, J. "Behavioral Assessment and Treatment of 'Organic' Behaviors in an Institutionalized Geriatric Patient." *International Journal of Behavioral Geriatrics* 1 (1983): 33–46.

Sands, D., and Suzuki, T. "Adult Day Care Alzheimer's Patients and Their Families." *Gerontologist* 23 (1983): 21–23.

United States Department of Health and Human Services. *Alzheimer's Disease: Report of the Secretary's Task Force on Alzheimer's Disease* (D.H.H.S. Publication No. ADM 84–1323). Washington, D.C.: U.S. Government Printing Office, 1984.

11

Treatment of Families of the Neurologically Impaired Aged

Joanne S. Lindoerfer

One of the saddest outcomes resulting from Alzheimer's disease is estrangement among family members. In some families, the stress associated with this disease results in bitter resentment.

In one family where the mother, Mrs. R., developed Alzheimer's disease we are provided with an illustration of how change in the affected member can put unique stresses on the functioning of the entire familial unit. While Mrs. R.'s husband was alive he would frequently mask the beginning signs of her dementia; this was done in ways that left others unaware of her memory deficits. However, when Mr. R. died, his wife's condition revealed itself to her relatives. A daughter became concerned when her mother telephoned in distress because she could not find her keys. Several minutes after hanging up, the mother repeated the call, having forgotten the earlier conversation. The daughter, unable to handle the patient's needs long-distance, and realizing that her mother was not functioning well on her own, arranged for Mrs. R. to enter a nursing home.

At this time, problems with the family became apparent. Mrs. R. expressed great unhappiness, especially to her sister, about living in the nursing home. After a time Mrs. R.'s sister insisted on taking Mrs. R. into her home. The decision was made against the daughter's wishes, and it demonstrated denial of the seriousness of the patient's problems. By so doing, the sister discounted the physical and emotional stress that had been experienced by the daughter. The sister, on the other hand, being about the same age as Mrs. R., may have felt personally threatened by the necessity of nursing home placement. These feelings of personal jeopardy on the part of the sister encouraged her denial of Mrs. R.'s decline.

When the realization struck the sister that she could not handle Mrs. R., she simply returned Mrs. R. to her own home, where she was still incapable of living alone. Conflict inevitably developed between the daughter and the sister. The daughter chose not to disrupt the lives of her husband and their children by either taking her mother into their home or by moving back to the city where Mrs. R. and her relatives lived. Long-buried guilt recurred as the daughter fretted over her decision to live hundreds of miles from her mother. The aunt blamed the daughter for not being "devoted enough" to her mother. A distinct coolness enveloped the extended family. At a time when mutual support would have been beneficial to all family members, an unfortunate emotional rift developed that prevented the family from functioning in an adaptive way.

In what follows, Joanne Lindoerfer, a clinical psychologist, explores common conflicts that occur within Alzheimer families and describes adaptive approaches that may be useful in mitigating or preventing family conflicts.

Dementia is a family problem. Alzheimer's disease is a stressful situation that disrupts the adaptive functioning of the family by changing the balance of long-standing relationships and exacerbating previous problems. A complete array of emotions emerges as the relatives struggle with the recognition that their family, as they know it, has irreversibly changed.

CONFLICTS WITHIN INDIVIDUAL CAREGIVERS

A partial catalog of caregiver and other family reactions consequent to dementia might include the following:

1. Anger with the patient for seeming to be stubborn, perversely and inconsistently "stupid," argumentative, unreasonable, and verbally and physically abusive.

2. Feelings of being overburdened with care of the patient, yet experiencing guilt over having those feelings.

3. Indecision about caring for the patient in the home as opposed to sending him or her to a long-term care facility such as a nursing home.

4. Frustration with the patient for behavior that he or she seemingly should be able to perform more competently, more quickly, or without constant reminders.

5. Embarrassment at the odd and often negative behaviors that the patient displays in front of others who do not understand, who stare, or who ask thoughtless questions.

6. The tendency of the caregiver to become isolated from social contacts and thus to feel lonely and alienated from normal society.

7. Ambivalent feelings of love for the individual who *was,* and desire to get away from the person who *is,* at least for a short respite (as well as guilt about the latter feeling).

8. Grief over the loss of the loved one (unfinished and confusing grief because the loved one is still present, if only in body).

9. Depression over the lost relationship and all the rewards that it entailed, be they warmth, security, sex, nurturing, companionship, intellectual stimulation, or any of the multitude of complicated interactions between intimate human beings.

10. Guilt about negative feelings and behaviors toward the patient in past years, and futile desire to atone to the patient, or irrational belief that the caregiver is responsible for the patient's condition.

11. Denial of the need for assistance in caring for the patient in an attempt to be everything for the patient.

12. Denial of feelings of hopelessness out of a fear that giving in will lead to a complete breakdown.

13. Total immersion in caregiving in order to avoid anger, guilt, and grief.

14. Guilt and anxiety about neglecting other family members, such as the nuclear family of the grown child, or the work responsibilities of the spouse or grown child.

15. No time to self.

16. Role engulfment and loss of self.

Compared to younger caregivers, older caregivers (usually spouses of the Alzheimer patients) are more likely to suffer adverse physical and psychological consequences from the stress of caregiving.

Perhaps more disturbing yet is the finding of a vicious cycle in which the stress reported by caregivers was reflected in their critical attitudes toward the patients, which in turn was associated with more destructive patient behaviors (threatening, physical abusiveness, wandering). These problematic behaviors, in their turn, led to more stress on the caregivers.

CONFLICT WITHIN FAMILIES

More complicated problems attendant to Alzheimer's disease involve open or hidden conflicts between two or more of the patient's relatives. Frequently, such conflicts have their roots in the past relationships of the individuals involved.

Open conflict in families of Alzheimer patients has been found to consist of three types of disagreements:

1. Overt disagreements about the definitions of Alzheimer's disease; for example, how serious the patient's memory loss is, and how much he or she is still able to do safely.

2. Expressed disagreements concerning family members' attitudes and behaviors toward the Alzheimer patient, such as not spending enough time with the patient, or not caring for the patient.

3. Expressed disagreements about family members' behavior and attitudes toward the primary caregiver; for example, not showing enough appreciation to the caregiver.

Hidden conflicts may involve:

1. Unstated disagreements about any of the above issues.

2. Unexpressed hard feelings about any of the above issues.

3. Unresolved tensions from earlier years, which the Alzheimer patients can no longer keep in check because of their impairment and changed roles in the families.

4. Tensions inherent in family members' changing relationships; for example, with the impairment of the patriarch, two or more of the grown children may compete for dominance within the extended family.

As examples of role changes within the family, consider that:

1. The patient may have been the confidante of family members.
2. The patient may have played the role of maintaining contact between, or peace among, other family members.
3. The patient simply may have been the one who managed the finances or took care of the house, and no one else can or will take his or her place.

Other dysfunctional patterns brought about because of the patient's impairment include:

1. Protection of certain family members from full knowledge and realization of the extent of the patient's impairment;
2. One family member voluntarily taking over the whole burden of caring for the patient, shouldering the guilt for the entire family, who avoid the patient.

Caregivers do, in fact, cite family conflict as a major problem, second only to the strain of caring for the Alzheimer patient. Compared to spousal caregivers, adult children caregivers are particularly likely to report open conflict, especially with their siblings. Although the absolute level of conflict was not reported to be high, research shows that conflict is associated with caregiver depression and anger. Depression is related to lack of support and appreciation, while anger is related to conflict over relatives' attitudes toward the patient.

On the other hand, good marital communication, strong family support (including emotional cohesiveness), role adaptability among family members, and ability to reframe or reinterpret family goals are associated with lowered stress and more satisfaction.

FAMILY BALANCE

It should be pointed out that, as in all systems, the family works to maintain a balance or *homeostasis.* Families have rules that define how their relationships should work. Examples of such rules include: (1) there should never be open conflict between two members of the family, or (2) no one should ever challenge the father's opinions./"Homeostasis" refers to the tendency of the family to keep members' behavior in line, such that if one of the rules is about to be broken, other family members will behave in such a way that the rule does not get broken. If the rule is that no open conflict is allowed, one of the members may change the subject so that the two members about to begin arguing are distracted from their argument. Homeostasis in the family is thus maintained.

Demands for sudden or great change in the rules may result in responses in other family members that tend strongly to maintain the original homeostasis. That is, family members who oppose the change will enforce the old rules, distract the members who are attempting to change the rules, or in other ways work hard to maintain the old rules. Certain rules in families are not only hard-and-fast rules, they are also rules about which no one is allowed to speak openly.

For example, the rule against open conflict may include the corollary rule that one may not talk about prohibiting open conflict. It is a rule that members must deny having but which nevertheless exerts its effects on all family members. A rule against criticizing parents may seem naive on the surface, and so may be disavowed by family members if they are confronted with its existence. The rule may be rigidly enforced, however, by family members who rapidly change the subject when criticism gets dangerously close to expression.

Needless to say, such unspoken rules often exert a stronger influence because they are more difficult for family members to acknowledge, and therefore to change, when circumstances require change. Even rules that have no sanctions against their acknowledgment are often difficult for families to perceive. Family rules are developed gradually and informally during the family's formation. Thus the rules are outside the awareness of the members because they have formed the backdrop of the relationships for many years, perhaps since before most members were born.

In certain more rigid families, rules are even more difficult to change than they are in other families. Necessary changes are met with inflexible opposition, or verbal distractions or other distractions, such as mental or physical illness or behavioral disorder.

SYSTEM FUNCTIONING IN FAMILIES OF NEUROLOGICALLY IMPAIRED INDIVIDUALS

Rigid rules and their enforcement can have the effect of stunting the growth and development of the individual or of separate subsystems in the family. Occasionally, unexpected circumstances occur (such as a family member developing dementia) that subtly or obviously change family behavior and put stress on its functioning. If family rules and the need for unbroken family homeostasis around unchanged rules prevent individuals or subsystems from performing new, more adaptive behaviors, those family members will experience distress.

Probably the most obvious change that takes place when a family member develops dementia is that the individual can no longer perform certain functions that he or she had always taken care of before. For example, a married couple may have originally agreed that the wife would take care of the cooking and cleaning, while the husband earned the living. If the wife develops dementia, she may no longer be able to cook safely, and the husband may have to take over her role as cook in the family. Besides feeling overburdened with the extra responsibility, the new cook may not want to see himself in the nurturing, "feminine" role of cooking, anymore than the afflicted wife may enjoy giving up her role. Conflict may and probably will arise in such a situation.

Conversely, if the husband is afflicted, then the wife, who may have enjoyed being dependent—the person cared for by a strong husband who made decisions about their financial dealings, living situation, activities, and the like—may strongly resist and be very unhappy in her new role as decision-maker when the husband is unable to do so. On the other hand, she may see the need and want to step into the decision-making role, but her children may resist having her in that position or may avoid seeing its necessity by failing to see evidence of their father's decline. Grown children may take sides in their parents' conflict over who should have certain responsibilities following cognitive decline.

Perhaps the caregiver is one of the children who, like all children, had a particular relationship with each of his or her parents. One of the rules in the relationship between a daughter and her mother, for instance, may have been that the daughter would be the mother's favorite, and she would always take care of her mother. When the mother then develops the very disabling symptoms of Alzheimer's disease, the daughter feels bound to her unspoken promise, the implications of which (in time and energy) she had not fully appreciated. The daughter may herself be torn between a desire to live up to the early rules of the relationship with her mother, and an equally compelling desire to live her own life. Circumstances have changed since she was younger and at home, and even since her mother became demented.

Conflicts between children in the family may have their roots in early sibling rivalries. One common pattern in families is to assign one child the role of "parental child"—that is, one child, typically the oldest, is sometimes given the task of being in charge of the other children in the parents' absence. That assignment may lead to resentment on the part of the other siblings. In addition, it may result in conflict when the parental child is reassigned the role of child upon the parents' return home. Such conflicts as these could carry over into adulthood and once again result in problems when one of the parents requires help from the children as the symptoms of a dementing illness unfold. In this case, siblings may criticize one another unfairly over expressing feelings about the demented parent or his or her treatment, or they may get into arguments concerning living arrangements.

Grown children may become uneasy when a parent is no longer able to continue the role of wiser, older adult, or they may feel guilty about challenging that role when they were adolescents and pushing for independence from the family unit. Unacknowledged and unaccepted feelings lead individuals to do things that they would not otherwise do, often to their own detriment and to the detriment of others. For example, guilt may lead a person to overcompensate. In a case where dementia is a problem, the guilt-ridden caregiver may become overinvolved in caring for the afflicted family member and neglect personal needs and responsibilities, which may result in not allowing the patient to do what he or she is still capable of doing. In fact, it has been found that when the caregiver was emotionally overinvolved with the patient, such that he or she overprotected the patient, there was an increase in negative patient behaviors such as anger, abusiveness, and paranoiac hiding of items. These behaviors in turn created more stress for the caregiver.

A common problem is the unwritten family rule that "conflict should never be open," or "negative feelings should never be expressed." Even in the best of circumstances, caregivers experience negative feelings on occasion during the arduous task of caring for the demented patient. While such feelings might not be expressed to the patient, it is best for the caregiver's emotional adjustment if they can be expressed to someone who is both accepting and understanding. Support groups of Alzheimer's relatives can be very helpful. It is important, however, for family members to learn to accept the feelings of their relatives and to express their own, even if no objective changes can be made in the family situation. Often the ability to express feelings leads to a heightened awareness in other family members, who might then suggest creative changes in care arrangements thus alleviating, to some extent, the burdens of the primary caregiver. For instance, if the healthy husband of an Alzheimer patient can express to his children his need for female companionship without risking their censure, he may feel freer to expand his social horizons and redevelop a side of himself that would otherwise be suppressed, possibly with rather severe consequences for his own well-being (e.g., depression).

FAMILY TREATMENT

What is family therapy? There are many different models of treatment for families in distress, and it is beyond the scope of this chapter to cover them in detail.

In most models of family therapy, all the members of a nuclear family are seen in a group session with one or two therapists or counselors. In some models, only one or two members may be seen, and the treatment is considered to be family therapy because the focus of discussion is on family relationships. At times, members of the extended family may also be involved in treatment, especially if they are closely concerned with the problems, as is often the case in families where there is neurological impairment of one of the older members. Treatment sessions are typically held weekly for ninety minutes, although they may be spaced more widely apart. In one model, families are brought in for an initial two-day treatment session and then brought back several weeks or months later to follow up on the treatment and to make further interventions if necessary. This is a useful model for families where members are spread over a wide geographical area.

In most models, family relationships are treated, rather than any one individual in the family, although frequently one person is the identified patient. In the family with a neurologically impaired member, the other members may define the demented individual as the patient or they may define one of the other family members as the dissatisfied one, i.e., the problem for everyone else. On the other hand, the family may come into treatment all acknowledging their distress, and ask for coping skills. In the early stages of treating families with a neurologically impaired member, the interventions may involve education about expectations of the impaired person, prognosis, and coping skills. However, treatment may need to go beyond education in order to maximize the well-being of both the family and the demented patient.

According to one model of family therapy, inappropriate behavior patterns are the result of family members' oversensitivity to and compliance with one another's needs and wishes to the detriment of their own development as individuals. Therapy sessions seek to demonstrate such entanglements. For example, some grown children may cope with a demented mother by avoiding her, while one daughter may respond to her brothers' and sisters' uninvolvement by becoming totally involved in caring for the mother, even to the point of neglecting her own nuclear family (i.e., her husband and children). She may resent her siblings' lack of involvement at the same time that they feel guilty about abandoning their sister and their mother. Or, more subtly, the caregiver may shield the other family members from discovering the extent of their relative's impairment, protecting them from a fact that they do not want to face. As a result, the caregiver prohibits herself from confiding in others about her feelings or asking for relief from her duties, and/or the rest of the family criticizes her when she does complain because they believe there is so little to complain about.

Family treatment would consist of demonstrating such patterns of protection, thereby helping family members to perceive their own feelings and roles in creating and maintaining such patterns. Therapy consists of helping family members to gain insight into maladaptive entanglements and to develop new, more adaptive patterns.

In another treatment model, families are viewed as having problems because they do not communicate straightforwardly, often using complicated communication patterns to maintain control over other family members. For example, one rather uninvolved member of a family may criticize the caregiver for discussing the possibility of putting the impaired member into a nursing home, the implication being that the caregiver does not love the patient. This may be an effort to handle personal guilt about abandoning the family member by attempting to keep the patient in the caregiver's home. Therapists may attempt to change levels of communication to more straightforward patterns by showing the family how to communicate well. Then again, therapists may engineer changes in one person's behavior that will automatically change the whole family's way of communicating.

Yet a third treatment model examines the family members' *ways* of communicating rather than *what* they communicate to each other. For example, members of the family may communicate only with each other, rather than with nonmembers, as in the case of a family that will not allow its members to let outsiders know about its problems, even when there is a desperate need for expert help. Yet the family itself may not ever resolve the problem(s), so that one or more of the members eventually feels great distress. Such a family would be said to be too *enmeshed* or intertwined with one another and too separated from the rest of the world. Certain particularly troubled families have been found to *avoid* seeking outside help with problems revolving around caring for an Alzheimer patient.

Therapy within such a framework involves helping the family to restructure itself to deal more effectively with the current situation, bringing in outside help if necessary. If the family is not enmeshed, but disengaged (that is, not sensitive enough to each other's communications), members may need help to restructure their relationships to be closer. Typically the therapist helps the family to change by engaging in exercises that give them practice in seeing current ways of communicating and in using new patterns of communication. For instance, the barriers between two subsystems may be too rigid for messages to pass across, so the therapist may ask one of the members to sit next to another member and to address him or her directly.

Studies have not uniformly shown family counseling to be successful in alleviating problems associated with caring for Alzheimer patients. For instance, family counseling focused on problem solving has sometimes yielded poor results. However, at least one study reported the success of family counseling in which the caregivers were taught to communicate their needs and the family to listen sensitively and to give emotional as well as practical support.

CONCLUSION

In summary, Alzheimer's disease and other neurological impairments are frequently very stressful for individual family members, whether they are involved as primary caregivers or only in caring for the patient on an occasional basis. Many of the stresses can be the result of family patterns of interrelating that may not be efficient or effective in coping with the previously unforeseen and possibly devastating consequences of neurological impairment. Families have patterns of relating that are formed in response to their developing needs and may or may not be useful in dealing with any given situation. Family therapy may be helpful in changing some of the detrimental patterns.

SUGGESTED READINGS

Barnes, R. F., Raskind, M. A., Scott, M., and Murphy, C. "Problems of Families Caring for Alzheimer Patients: Use of a Support Group." *Journal of the American Geriatric Society* 29 (1981): 80–85.

Goldenberg, I., and Goldenberg, H. *Family Therapy: An Overview.* Monterey, Calif.: Brooks/Cole Publishing Company, 1980.

Hinrichsen, G. A., and Niederehe, G. "Dementia Management Strategies and Adjustment of Family Members of Older Patients." *Gerontologist* 34 (1994): 95–102.

Hooker, K., Frazier, L. D., and Monahan, D. J. "Personality and Coping among Caregivers of Spouses with Dementia." *Gerontologist* 34 (1994): 386–92.

Knight, B. G., Lutzky, S. M., and Macotsky-Urban, F. M. "A Meta-analytic Review of Interventions for Caregiver Distress: Recommendations for Future Research." *Gerontologist* 33 (1993): 240–48.

Lazarus, L. W., Stafford, B., Cooper, K., Cohler, B., and Dysken, M. "A Pilot Study of an Alzheimer Patient's Relatives Discussion Group." *Gerontologist* 21 (1981): 353–58.

Mace, N. L., and Rabins, P. V. *The Thirty-Six Hour Day.* Baltimore: Johns Hopkins University Press, 1981.

Macera, C. A., Eaker, E. D., Jannarone, R. J., Davis, D. R., and Stoskopf, C. H. "The Association of Positive and Negative Events with Depressive Symptomatology among Caregivers." *International Journal of Aging and Human Development* 36 (1993): 75–80.

Maxey, L. B. "Therapeutic Interaction with Families of the Confused Elderly." In *Confusion: Prevention and Care,* edited by M. O. Wolanin and L. R. F. Phillips. St. Louis: C. V. Mosby Company, 1981.

Mittleman, M. S., Ferris, S. H., Teinberg, G., Shulman, E., Mackell, J. A., Ambinder, A., and Cohen, J. "An Intervention That Delays Institutionalization of Alzheimer's Disease Patients: Treatment of Spouse-caregivers." *Gerontologist* 33 (1993): 730–40.

Rankin, E. D., Haut, M. W., and Keefover, R. W. "Clinical Assessment of Family Caregivers in Dementia." *Gerontologist* 32 (1992): 813–21.

Schmidt, G. L., and Keyes, B. "Group Psychotherapy with Family Caregivers of Demented Patients." *Gerontologist* 25 (1985): 347–50.

Scott, J. P., McKenzie, P. N., Slack, D., and Hutton, J. T. "Families of Alzheimer's Victims: Family Support to Caregivers." *Journal of the American Geriatric Society* 34 (1986): 348–54.

Semple, S. J. "Conflict in Alzheimer's Caregiving Families: Its Dimensions and Consequences." *Gerontologist* 32 (1992): 648–55.

Skaff, M. M., and Pearlin, L. I. "Caregiving: Role Engulfment and the Loss of Self." *Gerontologist* 32 (1992): 656–64.

Smyth, K. A., and Harris, P. B. "Using Telecomputing to Provide Information and Support to Caregivers of Persons with Dementia." *Gerontologist* 33 (1993): 123–27.

Vitaliano, P. P., Young, H. M., Russo, J., Romano, J., and Magana-Amato, A. "Does Expressed Emotion in Spouses Predict Subsequent Problems among Care Recipients with Alzheimer's Disease?" *Journal of Gerontology: Psychological Sciences* 48 (1993): 202–209.

Williamson, G. M., and Schulz, R. "Coping with Specific Stressors in Alzheimer's Disease Caregiving." *Gerontologist* 33 (1993): 747–55.

Zarit, S. H., Orr, N. K., and Zarit, J. M. *The Hidden Victims of Alzheimer's Disease: Families under Stress.* New York: New York University Press, 1985.

12

What a Support Group Can Provide for Alzheimer Families

Beverly Smythia

This chapter is a moving story of a woman thrust into the role of caregiver. It is the story of a woman, perhaps like you, who came home one day from the doctor's office after learning that her life would soon become very different, but without much understanding of what to expect.

Mrs. Smythia and her family experienced the anger, frustration, and fears that most Alzheimer families face, but this particular family mobilized their strong feelings and put them into action. As a result of their efforts, in combination with other dedicated families in their community, a dynamic support group developed where none had existed before. This chapter not only provides inspiration, but also important ideas on how a support group can benefit its members.

At the age of thirty-two, I became a victim of Alzheimer's disease. My husband and our three children—then aged five, two, and six months—also became victims. No, we were not diagnosed as having the disease, but my husband's mother, Margaret, was. We became her caregivers, and we were to become victims as much as she. Our lives were drastically changed the day my mother-in-law came to live with us. I will tell the story of how we became caregivers, not because our story is unique, but because it is so common. What happened to us and the emotions we felt have happened to millions of other caregivers. I hope that a better understanding of these circumstances will underscore the need for support groups and support services to help Alzheimer families cope with their situations.

We had known there was something wrong with Mom for a long time. In the beginning, she also realized that something terrible was happening. At the time of their respective deaths, Margaret's mother and grandmother had both suffered from *senile dementia*. Mom feared that she, too, was becoming *senile*. She talked to her husband and to us about it; she even discussed it with her doctor. None of us knew anything about Alzheimer's disease. We told Mom not to worry. After all, she was a healthy woman in her fifties who had watched her diet. How could she possibly have "hardening of the arteries"? So Mom worried, and we reassured. But after a while, she stopped worrying. In fact, she denied being forgetful when she clearly was. That is when we began to worry.

At the time of this crisis, Mom lived 400 miles from us and was married to a very nice but older man. Both had been widowed and had married more for companionship than for love. Now, however, Mom was not a very good companion, and her husband was not able to carry her responsibilities as well as his own. He let us know that he wanted Margaret to live with us. He was making plans to leave her. Within a week, Mom had moved into our three-bedroom home. Soon after the move, Mom and Dad were divorced. It was not long thereafter that Mom was diagnosed as having Alzheimer's disease.

Becoming a parent to a parent is one of life's saddest and most difficult experiences. It is even more traumatic when the parent has Alzheimer's disease. Mom grieved so much after she came to live with us. She could not fully comprehend what was happening. Nor could she understand why her husband had rejected her and had wanted a divorce. She didn't want to live with us; she wanted to be in her own home, in her own church, with her own friends. She rejected our efforts to help her. A very proud and independent woman, she resented being taken away from her home. Day after day we explained why she was living with us. Day after day she cried, longing to go home.

I also grieved. I longed for the simple, uncomplicated life our family had enjoyed before becoming caregivers. I cried. I cried for what was happening to my sweet mother-in-law and for how I felt having to tell her time after time that she could not go home. I cried from the feeling of not having any control over my life. Alzheimer's disease had taken over my own life and had destroyed my freedom. I cried for the future. After reading the book *The Thirty-Six Hour Day* for the first time, I was terrified. For the first time I realized what Mom would become and what our future as caregivers would become. The greatest unspeakable fear concerned my husband and my children. Since Alzheimer's disease tended to develop in his family, would he become a victim too? I would look at my three beautiful children, so full of life and so bright, and wonder if their lives would end in a mindless state of dementia. It was as if a monster lived in our future, waiting to devour the people I loved more than life itself. How could I be certain that a cure would be found in time? I couldn't.

After weeks of carrying these burdens, I decided I could no longer continue along this path of self-pity and depression. I knew that if I was to survive, I would have to fight back. I had read about support groups, but there were none in our area, nor did I know another person who might be interested in a support group. But I knew there must be others like myself who needed to talk to someone who was also a caregiver. I had been frustrated by the lack of readily available information about the disease. Perhaps a group of caregivers could share information. After thoroughly discussing the possibilities with my husband, we decided to start our own support group. It was the first positive step we had taken since our family had become caregivers. For the first time, we felt that something good could come from our misfortune, something that would bring meaning to our struggle against this disease.

DEVELOPING A SUPPORT GROUP

Developing a support group takes planning and commitment from the organizers. The first step we took to create our group was to contact the Alzheimer's Association[1] for information on the disease and on how to start a group. The association was very encouraging and supportive of our efforts. They continued to nurture us until we were able to become a full chapter of the Alzheimer's Association. Since the beginning of our support group, the network of chapters of the Alzheimer's Association has grown tremendously and now stretches across the country. These chapters offer a wealth of information, training, and resources to anyone wishing to start a support group.

I'll never forget the first meeting of our support group. To my surprise there were twenty-six caregivers in attendance. Needless to say, we were very glad to meet each other. For some, it was the first time to talk to other caregivers, people who could really understand how it felt to see a

---

1. Alzheimer's Association, 919 North Michigan Avenue, Suite 1000, Chicago, IL 60611–1676; (800) 272–3900

loved one slowly slip away. For the first time, we knew we were not alone in our feelings. Our emotions of grief, anger, frustration, depression, and guilt were shared by others. We cried with each other and laughed at situations that could not be told even to friends, because they would not understand. From that day on, we knew we had brothers and sisters, of all ages and circumstances, who were together in their support of one another against an invisible but very real foe. In a very dark and lonely night, each of us became a small light for the other.

In the beginning I had a very narrow concept of just what our group would do. I had a vision of ten or fifteen people sitting in a circle and discussing problems. Occasionally we would have a speaker. Imagine my surprise when our group grew so fast that my husband's computer had trouble keeping up with it. Everyone was hungry for information. I soon found that support groups do a lot more than sit around and discuss problems, although that remains an important part of each meeting. A good support group has many roles to play; each one is very important in our battle against Alzheimer's disease.

Emotional Support

The first and most important role is that of giving emotional support to caregivers. The support group provides a safe and supportive community through which caregivers can share their thoughts and concerns. It is precisely this role of helping the patient by helping the caregiver that the support group can do best; and by helping each other, we help ourselves. Knowing others who have faced similar circumstances with courage and grace is also a source of encouragement to individuals who are afraid of what inevitably lies ahead. They discover new belief in their own ability to follow through on this difficult task.

It is hard to describe the transformation I have witnessed in caregivers who come to a support meeting discouraged and depressed and leave uplifted and strengthened. I have come to believe that you cannot be in the presence of courageous people without some of their courage becoming an inspiration for your own spirit.

Education and Information

Another important role of the group is to educate the caregiver. We have found that better understanding of the disease leads to an improved ability to cope with the many stressful situations that the caregiver must face each day. With more knowledge the caregiver feels in control and therefore better able to deal with each new stage. At this stage of research, very little can be done to change the course of this relentless disease, but we can prepare ourselves to face the inevitable decline of our loved ones. Acceptance is not easy, but it is possible. It is made less painful when the caregiver is better informed.

Caregivers also find that there is much knowledge to be gained from each other that will never be found in a book. When discussing problems, a group of caregivers can often discover new and creative ways of problem solving. Living under circumstances can many times cause caregivers to lose perspective of their situation. Talking a problem over with others helps them to see new ways of dealing with difficult situations. Once caregivers begin to think creatively, they are often better able to cope with new situations as they arise. The day-to-day tips that caregivers share with each other is an invaluable resource of the support group.

The support group also directs its members to community resources. Some groups develop resources of its own for use by its members. In most areas, there are few community services designed specifically for Alzheimer families, but there are some general resources that families can use if they meet the qualifications. The problem is that most families have no idea what resources are available and how the various systems work. The support group cannot possibly know every service in the community, nor can we counsel every family in need. Our job, however, is to know the agencies that can provide guidance through available social service systems. The Area Agencies on Aging can be valuable sources of information (see chapter 13). Working with a professional social worker through such an agency, families are guided to state and federal services for which they qualify.

Advocacy

Another major role of support groups is advocacy. The public has finally become aware of Alzheimer's disease, however, this does not mean that the problems Alzheimer families face in a system that is unresponsive to caregiver needs are fully understood. Caregivers are frustrated by widespread ignorance and neglect of their problems. It does not take long for the members of an independent support group to realize that the root of many problems can be found in local, state, and federal governments, all of which are largely unaware of the needs of caregiver families. Upon this realization, a support group may conclude, as our group surely did, that there is strength in numbers and that joining the Alzheimer's Association was the most practical course of action. The Alzheimer's Association is the organization leading the way for Alzheimer's disease advocacy at the national and state levels. Locally, the support group becomes an advocate by presenting speakers for community organizations, writing letters, and discussing problems with neighbors. Each caregiver can become an advocate in some form.

Special Projects

Many support groups discover that special projects are well worth their time and effort. Projects can involve fundraising, education, advocacy, or patient and family services. There are several ways they can be beneficial. Special events offer opportunities for media coverage which draws attention to the services the group provides and also furthers public awareness. Projects can give caregivers the opportunity to feel they are taking an active role in battling Alzheimer's. They are able to see themselves as a small part of a much bigger picture. For groups associated with the Alzheimer's Association, local support groups are offered the opportunity to take part in their chapter programs and projects as well as nationwide activities. Knowing your efforts are bringing about change can help caregivers to feel more empowered and less of a victim of this cruel disease.

CHALLENGE FOR THE FUTURE

Much has changed since I first became involved with a support group. There is much more public awareness about Alzheimer's and because of this, families generally are getting the diagnosis in the earlier stages of the disease. Consequently, their need for support and services lasts a greater of length of time. As this trend continues, there will be a need for more groups such as groups for early stages, male/female caregivers, adult children, children and teenagers, cultural specific, long-distance caregivers, and, most important of all, individuals diagnosed with the disease. The list of specialized groups is endless depending on the needs of the community. It is clear that as our population ages and more people are diagnosed at earlier times, the need for a variety of support groups will be ever increasing.

An important role of caregivers is that of advocate for the person with Alzheimer's disease. From dealing with medical, legal, and financial concerns to talking to state and federal officials for increased services, the victims of Alzheimer's disease depend on their families and friends to speak for them. Caregivers are the voice for those who no longer can speak for themselves. Through support groups, caregivers will receive the knowledge and resources needed to carry out this difficult task.

There is currently a great debate over the future of the health care system in our nation. All agree that changes must be made for Medicare and Medicaid to survive in the coming years. What is troubling about the debate is that there is no assurance these changes will bring about a better system of long-term care that is needed for families caring for those with Alzheimer's. In fact, there is the strong possibility that much of the progress that has been achieved over the past ten years toward unproved services and help for families may be wiped away. It is the responsibility of groups and caregivers to not only be aware but also be involved in this debate. We must call upon our nation's leaders to make policies that are compassionate and caring as well as fiscally sound.

CONCLUSION

I have tried to provide a better understanding of why support groups are needed, the role that support groups play, and what I believe will be the major challenges for the future of these groups. It is essential that the public and those in positions of power empathize with the emotions that caregivers face daily. Caregivers are in a *no win* situation. They know there are no "easy" or "best" solutions to the financial and emotional problems they face. The social and political system they have believed in and supported all their lives offers little help in their time of need. Most face the unkindest situation life can offer—that of hoping their loved ones would die before resources run so low that they can no longer be cared for properly. Their lives are filled with grief, frustration, loneliness, stress, and disappointment, yet I have never met people of such devotion and determination, whose overwhelming desire is to provide properly for their loved ones. I find it ironic that in a society whose members thrive on instant self-gratification, there are caregivers who sacrifice all and continue to love, even when their loved ones are only a distorted shell of their former selves.

I have been inspired by the love and devotion of the caregivers. They are today's unsung heroes. Their courage and spirit represent all that Americans have traditionally valued, and yet they are treated so callously and indifferently by our society. Surely they deserve better.

I said at the beginning that I had a vision of a monster in my family's future, waiting to devour all of us. Well, the monster is still there, but it is much smaller now. My fear of the monster has been replaced by anger and determination to see this disease eradicated. I hope others will have these same feelings toward this devastator of minds and souls, and will join our battle to see that this generation will be the last to suffer and to die from Alzheimer's disease. The monster can be slain, but it will take many swords fighting together.

13

Support Services for Alzheimer Victims and Their Caregivers

Virginia A. Seelbach and Wayne C. Seelbach

As a society we must determine what our ethical responsibility is to those whose physical and mental impairments make it impossible for them to provide for themselves. Many government agencies have been created in an effort to address this responsibility but, as many Alzheimer families have found, the resources available at this time are limited.

Is it necessary that a family be reduced to poverty before we, as a society, are willing to assist? One family that we interviewed had been forced to divorce in order to obtain the benefits necessary to maintain their household and still meet the health care expenses. Homes are frequently sold and retirement benefits are quickly exhausted. These issues are before our government and the wider public, but their resolution has not yet been accomplished.

Despite the acknowledged limitations in available support, there are programs designed to assist caregivers in their search for social services. Virginia A. Seelbach and Wayne C. Seelbach guide caregivers toward those who can help.

OVERVIEW OF SOCIAL SERVICES FOR THE AGED

The graying of America's population has been accompanied by a growing recognition of the special needs and problems that aging often produces for individuals, their families, and the larger society. Fortunately, our society is beginning to recognize the special difficulties that aging often presents, and has consequently established several sources of assistance for the elderly and their families. These services can be especially valuable in meeting many of the needs associated with Alzheimer's disease.

Of course, this neurological disease presents enormous problems for the afflicted as well as their caregivers. Beyond the questions concerning accurate diagnoses and medical treatment, there are significant social and personal issues that emerge and intensify throughout the course of the disease. What is the most appropriate and best way to deal with an affected loved one? How much should the family be reasonably expected to do in providing care? Is it a sign of family weakness or neglect to seek assistance from social service organizations? Exactly where can caregivers obtain assistance and sound advice concerning the care of the victim?

Unfortunately, many who could benefit from social support services often do not utilize them. There are several reasons for this underutilization. Some people view social services as "welfare" and avoid them at all cost. Others see care of the elderly, including Alzheimer victims, as exclusively a family responsibility. To seek or use "outside" assistance is seen as an acknowledgment of familial or personal weakness. There are still others who would avail themselves of social services if they were only aware that such services exist. This is perhaps the largest category of people in need, but who fail to obtain assistance that could lessen their burdens in caring for the impaired elderly.

Here we will direct attention to the existing and expanding social service and support networks that can provide assistance to elderly Alzheimer victims and their families in noninstitutional settings. Awareness and utilization of these services can ease the caregiving burden and improve the quality of life for all concerned. Some of these community-based services are primarily of benefit to the victim, while others are of more value to caregivers. Nevertheless, the benefits can be mutually reinforcing for victims, families, and the community.

SERVICES FOR THE ELDERLY

Chronological age is the sole criterion for many social services that may aid the Alzheimer victim. There are indeed a variety of community services for the elderly. While some programs serve only individuals older than a specified age, others may serve the spouse of a person who qualifies. Some senior citizen programs not only directly assist the person afflicted with a chronic dementing illness, but can also be of immense value to family caregivers and other family members. These services include such things as homemaker assistance, home health care, transportation assistance, home repair, nutrition programs, protective services, and income and property tax reductions. Some communities also offer free or sliding-fee legal aid, eye and dental care, and even free tax preparation assistance to people over sixty years of age. All persons who are over the age of sixty (whether or not they are victims of Alzheimer's disease) automatically qualify for the services provided through the Older Americans Act. Access to these services, which vary from community to community, can best be made through the local Area Agency on Aging, whose exact name may vary from state to state (e.g., Area Council on Aging or Office on Aging).

The local Area Agency on Aging is part of a nationwide network of federally funded offices that contract, advocate, and coordinate a vast collection of local services for persons over sixty years of age. These agencies perform an important "brokerage" function, i.e., they provide liaison activities linking people at various levels of need with the array of programs and services in a community.

A recent development at many local Area Agencies on Aging has been the provision of "case management" services for the elderly. The case management approach offers a "one-stop shopping" resource for meeting the multiple and varied needs of the elderly. Case management can be of immense value to victims of Alzheimer's disease. For example, after a complete assessment of the individual's social, medical, psychological, and economic condition, a case manager develops a comprehensive treatment plan. The case manager then monitors the client's progress and makes any necessary adjustments in the plan. Since social services consist of a broad range of often unrelated programs that revolve around a general goal of helping people get the things they need, the case management approach is especially useful in identifying and accessing each needed service while at the same time significantly reducing the frustrations that the social service bureaucracy frequently creates for victims and their caregivers.

SERVICES FOR VICTIMS

Although identified by Alois Alzheimer very early in this century, it is only in the last five to ten years that our society has begun to recognize the profoundly adverse effects Alzheimer's disease and various related disorders have on victims, their families, and their caregivers. Noninstitutional support services specifically for these victims are still in their infancy compared to the development of other types of multifaceted social services. Moreover, the nature and availability of such services vary a great deal from community to community and are often haphazard and incomplete.

A good example of the problems associated with providing care for victims of neurological impairments may be seen in the need for adult day care centers. Such centers need to have trained, professional personnel to provide various therapies, while a medical staff monitors the patient's health. The frequent turnover in day-care center clients, along with the high economic costs of providing such care, have combined to make such facilities unattractive and unprofitable for private enterprise. Compounding the problem is the fact that public awareness and support for such programs are slight. We are, however, beginning to see some signs of improvement in this regard. For example, some limited public funding is now being directed toward services for the neurologically impaired Alzheimer victim. Some insurance companies and investment organizations are presently studying and evaluating the possibilities for long-term care insurance and savings plans.

Because of the high costs associated with long-term care, some victims will qualify for social services based on a "means test," i.e., based on their income levels. Examples of these services include Supplemental Security Income (SSI), food stamps, utility bill assistance, free or discounted prescription drugs, Medicaid, homemaker services, home repair assistance, and a variety of other services that vary from state to state. Noteworthy, however, is the fact that such services are available to *anyone* whose income is below certain standards. Having a neurological impairment does not, in and of itself, secure financial assistance.

SERVICES FOR CAREGIVERS

Caregivers are the unheralded heroes of contemporary society. Not only do they give tirelessly of their time and energy, they also give of their economic resources. Financial assistance is often unavailable until the victim and the caregiver—especially if the caregiver is the victim's spouse—have exhausted their life savings and other economic assets. With the high costs of long-term care, economic destitution can occur quickly unless the victim resides in a state with liberal requirements regulating eligibility for economic assistance, such as Medicaid, or unless the victim qualifies for veteran's benefits. Even in these states the economic burdens of caregiving are heavy. Thus, it is important that caregivers be aware of all resources available to them and to the victims of the disease.

While often overlooked or underemphasized, services designed for caregivers are perhaps of as great a value as those directly intended for victims of Alzheimer's disease. The burden for caregivers is often quite stressful if not overwhelming. Respite from the stress of caregiving is a major concern for most of them. Short periods of relaxation enable caregivers to provide better service to their loved ones. A valuable service available in some communities is that of respite care, which allows caregivers a short but much needed time away from their caregiving duties. Family members are typically the resource used to provide respite for the primary caregiver. However, for a variety of reasons, this resource is sometimes unavailable. Relatives and friends, who often do not fully understand or comprehend the disease and its multiple ramifications, may avoid both the victim and caregiver and thus be unavailable to provide respite care. The fact that most Alzheimer victims are elderly means that they often have outlived many of their family members while, at the same time, the geographical mobility of our society has frequently placed younger family members at great distances from their elders. Thus, families may not always be available or able to provide respite for the primary caregiver. Community-based respite programs then become all the more valuable.

Most communities also provide some form of family counseling at reduced costs. Often there are educational programs and support groups as well. Support groups are especially beneficial in helping caregivers cope with the multiple stresses and in learning to deal with the physical and mental changes taking place with their loved one. Support groups have, moreover, come to be the organized voice and advocate for Alzheimer victims. These groups have made significant progress in making society aware of the many problems stemming from the disease. Their efforts are also beginning to show signs of success in channeling public funds toward research for the treatment and cure of Alzheimer's disease.

FINDING THE RIGHT SERVICES

It is essential to know how to access programs available for the neurologically impaired. Whenever problems emerge with any elderly person, the local Area Agency on Aging is the very best place to obtain initial information about services available in your community. While not a provider of direct services, it can very effectively serve a brokerage function of assessing needs and identifying appropriate and available resources. Since there is a local Area Agency on Aging available in *every* community in the United States, there is immediate access to information regarding community resources that can aid the elderly in general and victims of Alzheimer's disease in particular. To contact your Area Agency on Aging, check your telephone directory under "Area Agency on Aging" in the white pages, or "Social Services" in the yellow pages. Another valuable national resource for information and assistance is the Alzheimer's Disease and Related Disorders Association, which can be reached toll-free by dialing 1–800– 272–3900.

SUGGESTED READINGS

Brody, E. *Long-Term Care of Older People—A Practical Guide.* New York: Human Sciences Press, 1977.

Butler, R., and Lewis, M. *Aging and Mental Health.* St. Louis: C. V. Mosby Company, 1977.

Gwyther, L. *Care of Alzheimer's Patients: A Manual for Nursing Home Staff.* Washington, D.C.: Alzheimer's Disease and Related Disorders Association and the American Health Care Association, 1985.

Hale, G. *The Source Book for the Disabled.* New York: Paddington Press, 1979.

Heston, L., and White, J. *Dementia: A Practical Guide to Alzheimer's Disease and Related Illnesses.* New York: Freeman and Company, 1983.

Otten, J., and Shelley, F. *When Your Parents Grow Old.* New York: Funk and Wagnalls, 1976.

Silverstone, B., and Hyman, H. *You and Your Aging Parent.* New York: Pantheon, 1976.

14

Selecting a Nursing Home

Morris H. Craig and Raye Lynne Dippel

An elderly Hispanic man with Alzheimer's disease was placed in a nursing home. He was a model resident except for a single quirk that confused his caregivers: each morning this man would resist having his pajamas exchanged for daytime clothing. The institutional policy called for each resident to be neatly dressed during the day. This typically meek resident resisted the change of clothing and often became physically and verbally abusive.

Following an investigation by personnel in the nursing home, an explanation was found for this seemingly paradoxical behavior. This man was a proud individual, who was described as "macho" by his family. Even with dementia, the notion that female caregivers would undress and dress him was entirely unacceptable to him. Once this sensitivity was discovered a male attendant was assigned for purposes of dressing and no further outbursts occurred.

Selecting a nursing home that is responsive to the special needs of Alzheimer patients is the subject of this chapter.

THE NEED FOR NURSING HOME PLACEMENT

There will be a time in the life of the Alzheimer family when placement in a nursing home will arise as a serious consideration. The course of this horrendous disease is such that at some stage the patient's condition will deteriorate to the point at which family caregiving must be replaced by

161

the skilled care found in a nursing home. This usually happens after the family has gone through years of heartache, fear, frustration, financial burden, and emotional strain. Family members will have learned to live with a stranger who behaves in baffling ways. They will have seen their loved one change so much that the patient is no longer recognized as someone they once knew.

The decision to place the Alzheimer patient in a nursing home is not an easy one and can be an extremely traumatic experience for the family. To give the patient up to someone else can result in feelings of guilt, doubt, and a sense of failure. There can also be a feeling of relief to know that the patient will be receiving comprehensive care.

As soon as a diagnosis of Alzheimer's disease has been made, it is wise to begin planning for the care of the patient through all stages of the disease. Potential legal difficulties should be addressed (see chapter 15), financial planning should begin, and an active search for services available through the government and the community should be initiated. Although use of a nursing home facility may have been initially ruled out, it will still be of benefit to make inquiries into potential nursing homes early on to ensure that the best possible program is identified in the event that placement becomes necessary (see chapter 1). Some of the best programs have waiting lists for available openings; in some cases, the waiting period is one to two years. It is in the family's best interest to be well prepared for the possibility of nursing home placement. It is not uncommon for family members to make a pact with one another to "never" place Mom or Dad in a nursing home, only to realize late in the disease that they are unable to keep this promise. Finding a nursing home that will accept the Alzheimer patient can be a difficult task, and to find a home that will accept a patient who exhibits behavioral problems is even more difficult. Without proper preparation, the need for immediate nursing home placement could be a very stressful and disappointing experience.

Once the need for nursing home care has been established, the family should begin calling homes to determine financial arrangements, availability of beds, and the various levels of care offered. When this has been done, appointments should be made with facility administrators for tours to visit several facilities. For those homes being given serious consideration, repeat visits should be made at various times of the day and week to observe activities. The Nursing Home Visits Checklist provided at the end of this chapter may be useful in evaluating homes that the family is most interested in.

The family can become bewildered by the task of selecting the best nursing home for the patient. Too frequently such a choice has to be made on a trial-and-error basis. However, there is a selection process that can be helpful in reducing the trauma and uncertainty of finding the appropriate nursing home. That process will be discussed in the following sequence:

1. Cost
2. Nursing home philosophy
3. Standards and guidelines
4. Appearance and location
5. Staff expertise
6. Alzheimer's disease programs

COST

One of the first prerequisites to choosing a nursing home is to consider the financial aspects. Nursing homes can be expected to cost at least $1,500 per month. The cost of the nursing home facility will be determined in part by the level of care necessary for the patient. A physician orders the necessary services that determine the level of care needed.

It is important to inquire regarding the level of care offered by the nursing home facilities being considered. Some nursing homes provide only *intermediate* levels of care, which require medical supervision and assistance in health maintenance for patients with stabilized long-term illnesses. Until the terminal stage of Alzheimer's disease, when other medical problems such as pneumonia set in, intermediate care may be all that is needed.

There are nursing homes that provide only *skilled* levels of care, while others provide both intermediate and skilled care. The skilled level requires twenty-four-hour nursing, restorative therapies, or professional assistance; therefore, it is more expensive.

The care that nursing homes provide is basically paid for in three ways: private pay, Medicare, and Medicaid. *Private pay* refers to the total financial responsibility being shouldered by the patient and/or the family. Most private insurance policies do not cover custodial care and thus will not pay the nursing home expenses for an Alzheimer's patient. Some policies cover expenses accrued for hospice care when a patient is identified as having a terminal illness. The patient's insurance policies should be carefully reviewed to determine what services can be reimbursed. *Medicare,* on the other hand, is a government assistance program through the Social Security System for short-term, skilled-level care following hospitalization, while *Medicaid* provides government assistance for patients who have exhausted their resources or have low income levels and limited resources. Not all nursing homes will accept Medicare or Medicaid patients, since the home's participation in Medicare, Medicaid, or both programs is on a voluntary basis. Admission into a nursing home under the Medicaid program (Title XIX) is based on medical necessity, characterized by ongoing care, supervision, and client involvement with licensed nursing personnel. A primary diagnosis of Alzheimer's disease neither precludes nor ensures eligibility. Veterans may also qualify for benefits.

Medicaid

Alzheimer's disease has historically been considered a mental disorder rather than a physical illness and thus was not covered by Medicaid. There is currently a political movement to give official recognition to Alzheimer's disease as a physical disease. For an Alzheimer's patient to be determined eligible for Medicaid assistance with nursing facility (NF) expenses, medical eligibility must first be determined. The family's state Department of Human Services (DHS) will have application forms for the patient's physician to complete. The application form and medical record will be reviewed by a panel of physicians who determine medical necessity for NF care.

Financial eligibility will also be determined. For example, in Texas, at this time (1995), the patient must not have income greater than $1,374 per month and personal resources (bank accounts, IRA, money market funds, personal property—other than a homestead, etc.) must not exceed $2,000. When one spouse is in an NF and the other spouse remains at home, half of the couple's combined countable resources as of the month of nursing home entry (but a minimum of $14,964 and a maximum of $74,820) are protected for the spouse at home. This is called the protected resource amount (PRA). The institutionalized spouse becomes resource-eligible for Medicaid when the couple's combined countable resources are spent down to $2,000 in excess of the PRA.

Homesteads are exempt if the spouse/dependent relative will continue to live in the home. If the patient is living alone but signs a form indicating an intention to return to his home at some future date, then his home is also considered exempt. A Medicaid client in an NF, home and community-based waiver program, or demonstration project may place home property for sale without affecting eligibility. The value of the home property placed for sale (including life estates and remainder interests) is exempt until proceeds of the sale are received. If the client does not intend to return home, has no spouse/dependent relative living in the home, and the property has not been placed for sale, its equity value is a countable resource.

The community spouse's income is not considered in determining Medicaid eligibility. However, to the extent that the community spouse's monthly income is less than the minimum monthly maintenance needs allowance (currently $1,870.50), an income diversion may be made in the post-eligibility budget (the budget to determine the client's copayment toward the cost of NF care) from the institutionalized spouse to the community-based spouse to help supplement the latter's income up to the $1,870.50 limit.

In Texas, the patient's contribution toward the cost of NF care is calculated as follows: the client's total income less the $30 personal needs allowance, less the income diversion to the community-based spouse (if applicable), less the dependent allowance (if applicable), less deductions for incurred medical expenses (if applicable), less the home maintenance allowance (if applicable), less guardianship fees (if applicable), equals client's contribution (the "applied income").

Once eligibility is determined, the services provided include: hospitalization expenses, doctor's visits, and unlimited prescription drugs. It is also important to note that any eligible Medicaid recipient may receive up to fifty visits per year from a nurse or aide from an approved agency. For home health care, a written recommendation from a physician and approval from the Department of Human Services (DHS) are necessary. In Texas, DHS also has the community-based alternatives (CBA) program, which allows persons with a medical need to be in a nursing facility to receive Medicaid and nursing services at home as an alternative to institutionalization. The eligibility criteria for the CBA program are essentially the same as for the NF program.

Applications for Medicaid approval can be expected to take up to 45 days if the patient is sixty-five years of age or older, and up to 90 days if the patient is under age sixty-five. However, Medicaid coverage may be retroactive to the third month prior to the month in which the application was filed, if all eligibility criteria were met at that time. Early financial planning can help ensure that eligibility criteria are met. It may prove helpful to consult a financial planner and/or an attorney before making major financial changes.

Medicare

Medicare is available to anyone over sixty-five who is entitled to social security benefits, or those under age sixty-five who have been entitled to social security disability benefits for twenty-four months. To be eligible for supplemental security income (SSI) benefits in 1995, the combined income of both spouses who are living together in the same household cannot exceed $707 per month. For an individual living alone, the income limit is $478 per month.

Medicare will pay for up to 90 days of inpatient hospital care in any participating hospital during each benefit period. The deductible is $716 for the first 60 days, and an additional $179 a day for days 61-90. Medicare will pay for up to 100 days in a skilled nursing facility during each benefit period. Most nursing homes, however, are not skilled nursing facilities and are not certified by Medicare. Medicare pays all covered services for the first 20 days and all but $89.50 a day for up to 80 more days. Covered services include semiprivate room, all meals, drugs, medical supplies, regular nursing services, and rehabilitation services.

Home health care may also be paid by Medicare if the patient is confined to the home; there is no limit to the number of covered visits from part-time skilled nursing care, home health aides, occupational therapy, medical social services, and medical supplies and equipment. Medicare does not provide for custodial care, such as help with bathing, eating, and taking medicines, and does not cover most nursing home care. Doctors' services are provided for and include surgical services, diagnostic tests and X-rays, drugs that are presented as part of treatment and administered by a doctor or other health professional, and other benefits.

If questions arise regarding Medicare, call the local Social Security office. The phone number is listed in telephone directories under "Social Security Administration" or "U.S. Government." Local Social Security Administration offices will assist in making applications, in filing claims, and will answer any questions. "Medicare Survey Reports," which list homes that participate in the Medicare program, are also available at any local Social Security office.

Veterans Benefits

For current information on VA benefits and claims procedures contact a VA regional office. A call to 1–800–827–1000 from any location in the United States will connect you to a VA regional office. Counselors can answer questions about benefits eligibility and application procedures. They make referrals, when necessary, to other VA facilities, such as medical centers and national cemeteries.

VA medical center admissions offices are the immediate source for information regarding medical care eligibility and scheduling. They can provide information on all types of medical care, including nursing homes.

Veterans Nursing Home Care

Nursing care in VA or private nursing homes is provided for veterans who are not acutely ill and not in need of hospital care. The VA may, but is not mandated to, provide nursing home care if space and resources are available in VA facilities. Veterans who have a service-connected disability are given first priority for nursing home care. Veterans who may be provided nursing home care without an income eligibility assessment are: veterans with service-connected disability, veterans who were exposed to herbicides while serving in Vietnam, veterans exposed to ionizing radiation during atmospheric testing or in the occupation of Hiroshima and Nagasaki, veterans with a condition related to service in the Persian Gulf, former prisoners of war, veterans on VA pensions, veterans of the Mexican Border period or World War I, and veterans eligible for Medicaid.

Nonservice-connected veterans must submit an income eligibility assessment form, VA Form 10–10f, to determine whether they will be billed for nursing home care. Income assessment procedures are the same as for hospital care. Nursing home care may be authorized for nonservice-connected veterans whose income exceeds the income limit for hospital care, if the veteran agrees to pay the applicable copayment.

Veterans who need nursing home care may be transferred at VA expense to private nursing homes from VA medical centers, nursing homes, or domiciliaries. VA-authorized care normally may not be provided in excess of six months, except for veterans whose need for nursing home care is for a service-connected disability or for veterans who were hospitalized primarily for treatment of a service-connected disability.

Direct admission to private nursing homes at VA expense is limited to: (1) a veteran who requires nursing care for a service-connected disability after medical determination by VA, (2) a patient in an armed forces hospital who requires a protracted period of nursing care and who will become a veteran upon discharge from the armed forces, and (3) a veteran who had been discharged from a VA medical center and is receiving home health services from a VA medical center.

NURSING HOME PHILOSOPHY

The successful establishment and development of specialized nursing home services for Alzheimer patients is greatly influenced by the attitude of management and staff. A nursing home program will not extend beyond the shadow of its leaders. It is essential that the administrator be committed to developing better services for the Alzheimer patient.

Two schools of thought exist among nursing home administrators regarding separation of the Alzheimer patient from other patients. One approach is based on the concept that all Alzheimer patients should be grouped together in a separate unit. This arrangement has advantages from the standpoint of control, convenience, and better supervision. Such units can be designed to provide security and meet many of the specialized needs of the patient. Critics of this method quickly point out the need for those afflicted with Alzheimer's to socialize with other patients.

The second concept—nonsegregation of the Alzheimer patient—allows those suffering from Alzheimer's disease to be integrated into the regular program of the nursing home. Too frequently this arrangement does not provide adequately for the special needs of patients. The general trend is to establish separate units with specialized programs and trained staff. However, the success of Alzheimer programs will mainly be determined by the staff and how well they are trained. Nursing homes that seem to be the most effective are those where the staff believe that constructive things can be done for and with the Alzheimer patient. Families need to look for those homes that are flexible and open-minded in their approach to the patient. It is extremely important that the staff demonstrate understanding and affection toward Alzheimer patients. When visiting a nursing home, notice the interaction of the staff with the patients. Are patients introduced by name? Does the administration have someone on staff to show the facility, to point out special features and programs designed for Alzheimer patients, and to answer any questions that might arise? Are there specialized activity programs for Alzheimer patients?

Standards

Nursing homes must comply with state and local laws, whose standards have been developed for the care and protection of the patient. Each state has its own survey system for assuring that patients receive adequate care. Until recently the process focused on structural requirements more than on patient outcomes. This is beginning to change with new guidelines being developed to assess the quality of care provided by facilities. Standards of care include such things as ensuring that patients are receiving the specific diets ordered by their doctors, that grooming meets acceptable standards, and that medications are being dispensed properly. Accreditation reviews are very thorough, and generally take a full week to complete.

Part of the process of selecting a nursing home for Alzheimer patients involves determining that the prospective home complies with existing state regulations. Inquiries should also be made into what rating the home has been given, if a rating system exists in the caregiver's state. Is the home considered to be superior? These questions can be answered by the nursing home administrator.

When visiting a home, ask the administrator for the Bill of Rights for Residents of Nursing Homes, which all nursing homes are required to provide. The Bill of Rights should include the following principles:

1. The rights of Citizenship
2. The right to Dignity
3. The right to Privacy
4. The right to Personal Property
5. The right to Information
6. The right to Freedom
7. The right to Care
8. The right to Choose
9. The right to Residence
10. The right to Expression

Most states currently do not have separate standards and guidelines for the development of specialized nursing homes for Alzheimer patients. Some states are just beginning this task. The development of standards for Alzheimer facilities requires special consideration due to the uniqueness of the disease. The traditional programs will not suffice for the Alzheimer patient. There are different phases of the disease, and required treatment varies in each phase. A progressive program must be put in place, one that will allow for the various changes that take place in the patient's behavior.

APPEARANCE AND LOCATION

Structurally, a nursing home should look more like a home and less like a hospital. What effort is made to have familiar belongings in the patient's new home? Are patients permitted to have special pieces of furniture and bedcovers from their homes? Are pictures permitted on the wall? Many families believe that if a nursing home looks good and smells good, it will be a good facility. An attractive building in a beautiful location can certainly make a good impression. However, there are other factors to be considered in addition to the facility's appearance.

Is the nursing home safe for Alzheimer patients? Have provisions been made to prevent patients from walking away from the home and/or becoming lost? Wandering is considered to be a major problem in nursing homes; those located in heavy traffic areas present additional management problems and can be dangerous for the patients.

Will patients have easy access to the places they will need to go: restrooms, dining rooms, and activity rooms? Are there pictorial signs in easily observed places to facilitate the patient finding important places such as a restroom and perhaps his own room? For example, all restrooms might be painted orange with a picture of a toilet on the door. Perhaps the patient's picture and name in large letters might be on the door to his or her room. When confronted with a corridor of many doors all of which look alike, the Alzheimer patient can become quite confused and frustrated.

Good housekeeping practices are essential. The simple effort of removing wastepaper baskets and locking closets can prevent problems for the patient. It is important to ask if the patient will be allowed to live in one room for a long period of time or are frequent moves likely? Frequent changes in the environment result in difficult adjustments for the Alzheimer patient.

STAFF EXPERTISE

It should not be assumed that nursing homes will necessarily have adequate behavioral management programs. In fact some homes specifically forbid behavior modification despite evidence that such programs can offer very effective and humane means of managing behavior problems (see chapter 10). The absence of such programs generally indicates a lack of personnel trained in behavior modification principles; indeed, it is important that behavior modification programs be monitored by a licensed psychologist or other mental health professional specifically trained to administer them. Although some nursing homes are beginning to establish such programs and institute staff development needs, there remains a gap between what is being provided and what is needed. Many homes continue to depend on outside sources for assistance in providing specialized programs for their staff.

Practical and useful education programs are required for those staff members assigned to work with the Alzheimer patients. Coping with behavioral problems of Alzheimer patients requires skill, commitment, understanding, and patience. The staff must be willing to adjust to patient needs and change the programs and the environment to accommodate patient requirements rather than try to change the behavior patterns.

The lack of knowledge regarding the intellectual impairment caused by the disease and its various phases presents the staff with a great number of management problems. A basic fact that all staff should understand but often do not, is that Alzheimer's disease does impair memory, reasoning, judgment, and orientation—and it is irreversible. The nursing home staff also needs to be trained in how to handle such symptoms as depression, confusion, bewilderment, and emotional instability.

Training of staff members should be an ongoing process. This can be accomplished by using the various phases of the disease as guideposts for planning and conducting training sessions and in-house workshops. The staff needs to know what takes place in the life of the patient in the pre-diagnosis period. This provides an opportunity to link the patient's present behavior with previous patterns of behavior. For example, in one nursing home, the nurses were having a very difficult time getting one of their favorite patients to wear shoes. Much time and effort was expended getting Mr. R. to put on his shoes. When staff discussed this problem with his wife, it was learned that he *never* wore shoes at home throughout their forty years of marriage! Understanding previous behavior certainly facilitated their understanding of his present behavior.

Knowledge of the patients' general decline will help staff members better understand the drastic changes that have already taken place in the lifestyle of the patients and their family members. The last two phases, severe memory loss and total collapse of self-management skills, are usually the point where nursing home staff enter into the life of the patient. Special training regarding these crucial periods is essential if the staff is to understand and improve its skills in working with the patients, their families, and the larger community.

PROGRAMS

Long-term care statistics show that more than half the residents in a skilled nursing facility are diagnosed as having some form of dementia, many of the Alzheimer type. It is a challenge for a nursing home to design program activities that will meet the needs of the Alzheimer patients. Special planning and coordination is required to make dementia patients a part of things even though they cannot completely understand or participate fully.

It is important that nursing homes provide a smooth transition when moving the Alzheimer patient from the home to the facility. Some homes have a social worker or nurse specialist who conducts group sessions for family members. Family members can assist the transition by accompanying their loved one to the nursing home. It is helpful that a few familiar things accompany the patient to the nursing home.

Once the patient is established as a resident, the family should gain a clear understanding of what provisions exist for handling medical and nursing services. What arrangements exist for medical emergencies? The family will also want to know what types of social programs and rehabilitation services are available.

Most nursing homes will routinely develop individualized patient care plans. A care plan is a specific overview of the patient's strengths and weaknesses, specific objectives for patient self-management, and the staff assistance required to help the patient with daily activities. Such a plan calls for prioritizing activities on an individual basis. The care plan should also include documentation of what is to be done for the patient: when, how, and by whom.

The better Alzheimer programs are designed with the patient in mind. Special planning is given to exercise, social activity, privacy, and respect for personal rights. Exemplary programs designed specifically for Alzheimer patients may include any of the following:

1. Architectural and interior design planning to reduce visual ambiguity and to encourage independence (see chapter 4) by facilitating ease in identifying people, places, and time (see chapter 9): for example, pictorial signs to identify important areas, large wall clocks, and name tags for staff.

2. Secure wandering areas are important. What precautions have been made to ensure that the patient does not wander off? Alarms or bells on exit doors will alert staff that someone has left the facility. Since patients will frequently remove identification tags (such as those worn on the wrist), identifying labels sewn into clothes, or special articles that the patient is unable to take off, may facilitate identification and return of a lost patient.

3. Reality training, orientation therapy, and reminiscence therapy are excellent programs to encourage both social activity and orientation to the environment (see chapter 9).

4. Music therapy and art therapy are often provided to Alzheimer patients.

5. An exercise program is very important (see chapter 3).

6. Family education and support services will be included in the best programs.

7. Self-care (e.g., grooming, eating, and the like) will be encouraged by staff who are trained to break down tasks into manageable units and then assist only as needed. Frequently it is easier for the staff members to do something for the patient rather than allow the time for the individual to work through it. This, however, does not promote optimal levels of independence.

8. Good programs will provide a daily patient routine that is consistent and structured such that the patient is not left alone for long periods of time.

9. Good programs will encourage affectionate contact (e.g., patting hands, a hug or two, etc.) and as much social interaction with the staff as the patient is able to tolerate comfortably. The staff will

be encouraged to treat patients with respect, preserving their personal dignity.

10 Efforts will be made to ensure that the staff remains as constant as possible, avoiding nurses and aides having frequent shifts in the units that they serve.

11. A good program will invite family input regarding the patient's preferences and needs.

12. There should be regularly scheduled in-service training seminars on management of Alzheimer patients. (Staff turnover will be minimized by providing good training and by responding to the staff's emotional needs.)

13. The best programs will have on staff, or will work closely with, professionals who have been trained in behavior modification principles.

Volunteers can make a positive contribution to the patients' quality of life, particularly in providing help feeding those who need assistance. This type of service can be extremely helpful to both the patients and the staff.

Alzheimer patients require more direct care than other patients. This type of work is stressful and requires staff who can manage their own thoughts and feelings. Traditionally, a high turnover in staff has occurred in nursing homes; these rapid changes in personnel are hard on the patients and expensive for the facility. Nursing homes are becoming more alert to personnel needs. Staff members definitely need a release valve for their own frustrations and disappointments.

Problem Patients

The aggressive Alzheimer patient may be refused admission to a nursing home or may be asked to leave if the nursing staff is unable to manage. Nursing home aides are frequently female and may not be strong enough to manage large, aggressive patients. If aggression is likely to be a problem, this should be addressed to the nursing home administrator when the family is touring a prospective facility. Reliance on restraints to manage behavior is counterproductive. Although restraint may be needed on rare occasions, it is not an acceptable substitute for the proper management of behavior problems. Honesty with nursing home administrators regarding problems in managing the patient's behavior will lead to better care and an increased likelihood that the home will be able to manage the patient effectively.

In the event that a nursing home rejects a patient on grounds of behavior problems, search out other nursing homes whose staff may be better prepared to handle the problem behavior. It may become necessary to return the patient to the home and provide twenty-four-hour nursing care. Commitment to a state hospital may also be possible if it is determined that the patient is a danger to himself or others.

Although physical abuse is unlikely to occur in nursing homes, there are rare occasions when untrained personnel may react in kind to an aggressive response. If the family has any reason to believe that abuse is occurring, or may have occurred, concerns should be relayed to the nursing home administrators, who will address the problem. Families should be alert to neglect, which is another uncommon form of abuse. Most nursing homes make every effort to provide a safe, humane environment, but there are exceptions. Federal law now requires that each state have a State Nursing Home Ombudsman who investigates and resolves complaints on behalf of nursing home residents.

CONCLUSION

One of the greatest burdens for the family caregiver is the lack of knowledge of community resources and the ability to utilize these resources. In reality, the Alzheimer's disease care system has been a fragmented approach designed to function on a crisis basis. The needs of the patient and the family have been poorly understood and have received little societal attention. To further complicate the situation, confusing eligibility requirements make it difficult to identify available services. Preparation well in advance of need and a careful review of potential nursing homes may save families much grief. Mental health agencies, the Social Security Administration office, state Area Agencies on Aging (see chapter 13), and local support groups (see chapter 12) are much needed sources of valuable guidance.

APPENDIX
NURSING HOME VISITS CHECKLIST

Home A: _____

Home B: _____

Home C: _____

	Home A	Home B	Home C

LOCATION

1. Is the home close to family and friends? .... ( )   ( )   ( )

2. Is home on an expressway where the patient could wander off and get hurt?........................... ( )   ( )   ( )

LAYOUT

1. Do residents have places to put personal possessions?.. ( )   ( )   ( )

2. Is there adequate privacy in bathrooms and around the beds?... ( )   ( )   ( )

3. Are there places for private conversations with visitors?.. ( )   ( )   ( )

4. Are there handrails and grab bars in the halls and bathrooms?.. ( )   ( )   ( )

5. Are there sufficient smoke detectors and fire extinguishers? .... ( )   ( )   ( )

6. Are exits clearly marked and unobstructed?...... ( )   ( )   ( )

7. Are there call buttons for each bed and in the bathrooms?.. ( )   ( )   ( )

8. Is there additional heat available in the bathrooms?.. ( )   ( )   ( )

9. Does the home have a lounge for the residents? ( )   ( )   ( )

	Home A	Home B	Home C

10. Is there a safe, contained outdoor area for the patient to walk about?..................................... ( )   ( )   ( )

11. Are restrooms easily identifiable by pictorial signs?.. ( )   ( )   ( )

12. Do patients' rooms have easy access to lounges, restrooms, and cafeterias?................... ( )   ( )   ( )

13. Is furniture designed for ease in sitting, standing, and moving about?............................ ( )   ( )   ( )

14. Are patients' rooms marked for easy identification by each patient?............................ ( )   ( )   ( )

CLEANLINESS

1. Is the home reasonably free from unpleasant odors?... ( )   ( )   ( )

2. Is the home generally clean and orderly? .... ( )   ( )   ( )

3. Are employees clean and well groomed? .... ( )   ( )   ( )

4. Are patients clean and well groomed?.............. ( )   ( )   ( )

5. Are the bathrooms sanitary?............................. ( )   ( )   ( )

6. Is the kitchen clean? .... ( )   ( )   ( )

FOOD

1. Is the menu varied but with balanced, nutritious meals?.. ( )   ( )   ( )

2. Are special diets provided for residents who need them?... ( )   ( )   ( )

3. Are adequate between-meal and bedtime snacks provided?.. ( )   ( )   ( )

	Home A	Home B	Home C
4. Does the food taste good?	( )	( )	( )
5. Are serving sizes ample?	( )	( )	( )
6. Are second helpings available?	( )	( )	( )
7. Are Alzheimer patients encouraged to feed themselves when at all possible?	( )	( )	( )
8. Are Alzheimer patients fed by hand when they are no longer able to feed themselves?	( )	( )	( )

ATMOSPHERE

1. Is the home warm and cheerful?	( )	( )	( )
2. Are residents treated with dignity?	( )	( )	( )
3. Are the staff and administrators courteous, cheerful, and enthusiastic?	( )	( )	( )
4. Do staff members make eye contact with residents, speak clearly and loudly, and wait for residents' responses?	( )	( )	( )
5. Are residents treated with warmth and affection?	( )	( )	( )
6. Do staff members respond calmly and without anger toward emotional outbursts or noncompliance by Alzheimer patients?	( )	( )	( )

ADMINISTRATION

General

1. Is the home certified for Medicare?	( )	( )	( )
2. Is the home certified for Medicaid?	( )	( )	( )
3. Does the home have a current state license?	( )	( )	( )

	Home A	Home B	Home C
4. Does the administrator have a current state license?	( )	( )	( )
5. Are all costs clearly specified in terms of both amount *and* coverage? (Ask about extra costs for laundry, hairdressing, etc.)	( )	( )	( )
6. Are refunds available for unused services?	( )	( )	( )
7. Are there written procedures for handling residents' personal funds and valuables?	( )	( )	( )
8. Was a written statement of residents' rights provided to you?	( )	( )	( )
9. Under what circumstances can the home discharge a person, and how much notice must they give you?	___	___	___

Medical

1. Is a physician available at all times in case of emergency?	( )	( )	( )
2. Does the home have an agreement with a nearby hospital in case of an emergency?	( )	( )	( )
3. Are there established procedures for reporting to the family unusual incidents involving the resident?	( )	( )	( )
4. What is the health care staff-to-patient ratio on the various wings or floors?	___	___	___

Programs

1. Is there a special program designed for Alzheimer residents?	( )	( )	( )
2. Are there reality orientation exercises?	( )	( )	( )
3. Is reminiscent therapy provided?	( )	( )	( )

	Home A	Home B	Home C
4. Is there a daily exercise program?	( )	( )	( )
5. Are patients encouraged to provide for their own grooming when possible?	( )	( )	( )
6. Is there specific staff training for managing Alzheimer patients?	( )	( )	( )
7. Is there staff education regarding stages of Alzheimer's disease and expected symptoms?	( )	( )	( )
8. Is there a consultant or staff member trained in behavior modification principles?	( )	( )	( )
9. Are there family education and support services provided?	( )	( )	( )
10. Are family members invited to contribute to treatment planning?	( )	( )	( )

(Nursing Home Visits Checklist was modeled after a checklist provided by a Texas Attorney General's office pamphlet titled "Selecting a Nursing Home.")

SUGGESTED READINGS

Barrows, G., and Smith, P. *Aging, The Individual and Society,* 2d ed. St. Paul, Minn.: West Publishing Company, 1983.

Burke Rehabilitation Center. *Choosing a Nursing Home for the Person with Intellectual Loss.* 785 Mamaroneck Avenue, White Plains, New York 10805.

Morris, C. "Specific Behavior Problems in Nursing Homes—Alzheimer's Disease." Second Annual Conference, Working with the Aged, Lubbock, Texas, 1982.

Texas Department of Health. "Alzheimer's Disease Initiative Nursing Home Study." July, 1985.

15

Legal Considerations

J. Ray Hays

The author's parents recently were in a restaurant in the small town in north Georgia where they live. As dessert came, two men approached his parent's table. The elder of the two, always the Southern gentleman and ever gracious, complimented his mother on the way she was dressed, then turned to his father and said, "Now I want you to be sure and come by the office tomorrow and sign those papers. We've got to get them to court."

Such an interchange could occur anywhere. What is important about this event is that the man in question was an attorney by training but had not practiced law for at least ten years and had no business dealings with the author's father for even longer. The man was successful, being both diligent and smart in his dealings with the courts and clients. However, as he approached his retirement years he became neglectful of his personal appearance and some of his business dealings. He had struggled with alcohol abuse early in his life and had overcome this problem with the help of his law partners. When these new problems of attention to his personal care, business, and social relationships became evident, those who cared for him actively sought to resolve them. He was fortunate that he had business partners who would protect him from the consequences of neglect of important matters and a family who would intervene when needed. As his problems with memory progressed he gave up the practice of law, turned the care of his various business interests to others, and concentrated his efforts on the tasks of retirement.

Because of his children's knowledge and timely intervention, this was a success story for him and his family. However, without thoughtful care, planning, and a willingness to intervene by concerned family members the outcome could have been disastrous.

J. Ray Hays provides an overview of the legal issues that Alzheimer families need to be aware of to ensure that careful planning can be made well in advance of the need for legal intervention.

Families facing the difficulties of dealing with a relative who has Alzheimer's disease need to be aware of the protection and assistance they can obtain from the courts. This chapter reviews issues of guardianship, wills, commitment, and other legal matters related to care of the elderly or incompetent person. Families with specific legal problems should consult an attorney who deals with such issues. Elder law, wills, estates, and trusts are an emerging specialty in the law, and a family who takes the time to find competent assistance will be rewarded.

GUARDIANSHIP

About 15 percent of adults in the United States provide special care for sick relatives, many of whom are seriously ill or disabled. This is a significant public health problem and shows that those family members who care for persons with diseases such as Alzheimer's are not alone in their responsibilities. Society's concern in the form of legal expression has developed to deal with the problems of infirm persons.

Early in the course of Alzheimer's disease, the family should prepare for the patient's eventual decline in judgment by inquiring into procedures needed to obtain guardianship. These procedures vary from state to state, as does the extent of disability needed to warrant guardianship. A *guardian* is any person appointed to manage the person, property, or rights of an individual when proof is presented to the court that the individual is not competent to manage his or her own affairs.

In many states there are several types of guardianships that may be pursued when some intervention is needed with an infirm family member: (1) guardianship of the infirm person's estate, (2) guardianship of the person, which allows the family to intervene to protect the patient's health or welfare, and (3) a mixture of the other two types of guardianships.

Guardianship of the Estate

In a *guardianship of the estate* the alleged incompetent person must be shown to be incapable of managing his affairs, meaning that complete incompetence need not be shown. A lack of business sense, physical infirmity, or poor memory are, by themselves, not necessarily enough to warrant the imposition of a guardianship. The court will look to the person's total circumstances and then decide if a guardianship is needed. The totality of circumstances includes the size and complexity of the estate, and other factors that need to be examined. In Alzheimer's disease the extent of memory loss and rapid decline of personal care capability could prove to the court that an individual does not have the capacity to manage the affairs of daily life. If this is indicated, then the court will appoint a guardian.

Guardian of the Person

A *guardian of the person* is appointed when the individual under consideration is no longer capable of managing himself and must be placed under the care of others. This can occur in both chronic and acute disease situations: the individual is robbed of the capacity to make decisions, and others must make decisions for him. For example, before most medical procedures are performed, the patient must provide consent. Informed consent requires that the individual knowingly and willingly consents to the procedure after the risks and benefits are explained. When the patient is unable to understand the risks and benefits of the procedure, informed consent cannot be obtained and the procedure may not be performed. When this occurs, the physician or hospital may pursue the appointment of a guardian to provide substituted consent. In some jurisdictions, when an Alzheimer patient is unable to give informed consent the next-of-kin can provide it, with the assent of the patient.

A guardian may sometimes be limited in the ability to consent to care. For example, some states do not allow a guardian to consent to procedures such as electroshock therapy or discontinuing life-maintaining procedures. In such states it may be wise to execute a *durable power of attorney for health care* which will allow substituted consent to a full range of medical decisions even in the presence of incompetency of the patient.

ADVANCE DIRECTIVE

Advance directive is a euphemism for outlining what a patient wants done or not done to preserve life when there is a terminal illness or the patient is in a persistent vegetative state. The advance directive is a way of respecting the wishes of a patient without having to obtain a guardianship. By federal law such directives are required before admission to any inpatient facility. However, they must be executed by an individual who is competent. Patients with advanced Alzheimer's disease are not competent and would not be able to complete such a directive. In those circumstances a relative or other person previously indicated by the patient may execute an advance directive with the advice of the attending physician.

In the event that an individual has reached the terminal stage of an illness and the attending physician is considering an order not to resuscitate, an order to discontinue use of a respirator, or one to discontinue feeding the patient, the family is consulted. A guardian may be appointed to give an objective view of the situation, one that the family may not yet have grasped. This is an evolving area of the law, and we may well reach the point where the consent of a guardian is required before a "do not resuscitate" order is written for a patient. This procedure is used where no advance directive has been executed or there is no durable power of attorney for health care.

Who May Be a Guardian?

The court has a great deal of latitude in selecting a guardian. Those individuals who have the most interest in the welfare of the incompetent person are the court's first and most likely choices. In the absence of a family member or other close relative, the court will look to those who have some legitimate interest in becoming the guardian. In such case, family friends or attorneys frequently assume the role of guardian. Generally, a staff member of the administrative head of a treatment facility is not a good choice to be guardian. Such individuals have a less-than-objective involvement with the incompetent person, as each stands to gain monetarily so long as the patient continues to receive care. Such dual roles have an inherent conflict of interest and should be avoided.

What May a Guardian Do?

Guardians operate under a grant from the court to act in the incompetent person's interest, as if the person were deciding for himself. The powers of the guardian can be limited or complete, depending upon what the court decides is warranted by the patient's needs. Often the incompetent person is quite capable of managing many daily activities but is unable to cope with the pressures of financial matters; here the guardian may simply be a money manager. For example, the guardian may receive social security checks, pay rent and utilities bills, and so on. Daily care is left to the individual so long as he is able.

The guardian may only act to the extent that the limited grant of power from the court allows. Should a limited guardianship be obtained, the family or the guardian will have to return to court and request a broader range of power in the event that additional responsibilities need to be assumed by the guardian as the disease progresses.

POWER OF ATTORNEY AND TRUSTS

The *power of attorney* allows an individual to act through others; it permits the individual upon whom the power has been conferred by the court to make decisions pertaining to someone's real and personal property as though the true owner had so decided. Some states do not allow a power of attorney to continue after an individual becomes incompetent, while other states do if there is a provision in the power of attorney that authorizes its continuance even when the person becomes incapacitated.

Trusts offer another method through which an individual can permit others to assume partial or full control over financial matters. One or more persons can be named to manage their property, income-producing assets, bank accounts, and other financial matters. The use of a trust arrangement allows an individual to avoid an appointed guardian in the event that he becomes incapacitated. This is the ultimate form of pre-planning for the contingency of incapacity. To initiate a trust the family will require the services of an appropriate financial institution, such as a bank or trust company, as well as an attorney.

COMPETENCE TO MAKE A WILL

The capacity to make an effective will is a frequent subject of newspaper headlines both when a great deal of money is involved and when an unusual beneficiary is named. The family of an Alzheimer patient should consider obtaining a will when there is any type of estate, whether in the form of real or personal property, that would, under ordinary circumstances, pass to heirs. The life expectancy of an Alzheimer patient is much shorter than for healthy persons of the same age. If there is not already a will, the family should obtain one as early as possible. Obtaining a properly executed will may preclude some of the disputes among potential heirs which might otherwise occur.

Elements of Testamentary Capacity

The *law of testamentary capacity* is fairly straightforward with four elements that must be present. First, the person making the will, the testator, must have an understanding of the nature and extent of the property to be bequeathed. Second, the testator must be able to formulate a reasonable plan for the distribution of the property. Third, he must be able to understand the relationship between himself and the natural objects of his bounty, that is, those individuals who would ordinarily be in the mind of a person making a will. Fourth, the testator must be able to keep all these elements in mind at the time of execution of the will.

Adults are presumed to be capable of making a will unless proven otherwise. It must be shown by the person contesting a will that one or more of the required elements was missing or that some other factor was present thus rendering the will invalid. Perfect sanity is not required. Even an individual who was legally insane might be able to make a valid will if the four elements are present when the will was prepared. An individual who has been diagnosed as having Alzheimer's disease might still be capable of making a will during lucid periods when all the elements for testamentary competency are in mind at the same time. As with most diseases, the symptoms of Alzheimer's wax and wane in expression. The family should use those moments of lucidity to the patient's advantage by having a will executed.

PROBLEMS WITH WILL EXECUTION

There are at least two problems that could be used to defeat the executed will of an Alzheimer patient: insane delusions and undue influence.

Insane Delusions

An *insane delusion* is a belief held by an otherwise stable person who clings to it in spite of proof that most people would accept as compelling evidence that the belief is false. An example of an insane delusion might be the suspicion of a person who is convinced that his spouse is trying to poison him. Mild paranoid delusions are sometimes found in Alzheimer victims as they try to make sense of their increasingly confusing world. "Someone is hiding all of my shoes!" "Someone is taking my keys. I know I left them here." Such delusions would be problematic if the patient, while making a will, decided to cut his daughter off because someone had been hiding things from him.

Undue Influence

Individuals who have Alzheimer's disease are frequently unable to keep events or individuals in their minds for any length of time. They become creatures of the moment, acting on impulse or whim and influenced more than most by those who are near them at the time. This behavior makes them susceptible to the influence and domination of others. The result can be undue influence. For instance, a new acquaintance who does not have the patient's and family's best interests at heart may act to influence the patient in such a way that the patient suddenly alters his will, leaving his entire estate to the "friend." The pressure to make such a change may be constant and coercive in nature, an obvious attempt to take advantage of weakened reasoning.

Undue influence has been defined by one court as the exercise of control of one person over another so as to overcome the second person's free exercise of choice. A person of sound mind has the legal right to dispose of his property as he wishes. If family, friends, or organizations desire to contest a will that they perceive was written under undue influence, the burden is on those protesting the disposition of property under the terms of the will to prove that it was the product of such influence. Undue influence on testamentary capacity can be claimed when mental coercion is used by someone to influence the disposition of property. The crucial question is whether or not the individual was exercising a choice free of coercion when the will was prepared or whether the will of another person was substituted for that of the testator.

The old saying that an ounce of prevention is worth a pound of cure applies to wills. When an attorney believes that his client is seeking to dispose of property in a manner that might be contested by potential heirs, it is useful to have a psychiatrist or psychologist examine the testator at the time the will is executed. An affidavit could then be executed to the effect that the testator was examined by the expert for the purposes of establishing competence.

INVOLUNTARY CIVIL COMMITMENT

The family of an Alzheimer patient may pursue involuntary commitment to a state institution when the patient's behavior has become so disordered or disruptive that it becomes intolerable or unmanageable. Some nursing homes are unwilling to accept a patient who poses severe behavior problems and demonstrates a significant lack of personal care, as is sometimes the case with Alzheimer patients. For these reasons family members may want to consider the commitment process.

Each state has some provision for the involuntary commitment of individuals who are mentally disturbed. In most areas of the country community mental health centers provide families with advice regarding commitment procedures. In larger communities there are specialized courts and court personnel who deal exclusively with such problems. The local mental health association is generally a good source of information on such matters.

There are generally three requirements that must be met before an individual may be involuntarily committed, although these requirements may vary from state to state: (1) the individual must be determined to have a mental disorder, (2) he or she must require hospitalization (for example, the patient cannot manage in a less restrictive environment), and (3) the person is a danger to himself or others. There must be at least clear and convincing evidence of these three requirements, generally based on recent overt acts, before an individual may be committed.

During the 1970s there were several landmark judicial decisions related to the return of mentally impaired individuals to community facilities. These decisions dealt with the right to refuse treatment, the right to less restrictive alternatives to institutionalization, and the right to treatment.

Right to Treatment

Once an individual has been hospitalized, what must occur? What is the obligation of the state to provide treatment? The U.S. Supreme Court, in its decision of *Donaldson* v. *O'Connor,* stated that the right of society to involuntarily hospitalize a person who is not dangerous is based on a *quid pro quo.* The right to hospitalize rests on a responsibility to provide treatment. In Donaldson's fourteen years of hospitalization the court noted that all he received was "milieu therapy," which, in his case, consisted of sitting in a room filled with other persons who were deemed mentally ill. Without more evidence that treatment was being provided, the Supreme Court declared Donaldson was unjustly hospitalized and ordered his release. The basic premise of this case is that a patient who is hospitalized must be treated or released provided they represent no danger to themselves or others.

Right to Refuse Treatment

Once a patient has been hospitalized, what is the right of the patient to refuse treatment? The United States District Court of New Jersey, in the case of *Rennie* v. *Klein,* set a precedent for determining the conditions under which a psychiatric inpatient has the right to refuse treatment. John Rennie was an involuntary mental patient who, at the time of the hearing, had been admitted to psychiatric hospitals twelve times. Although involuntarily committed, he had never been declared incompetent. Rennie brought a civil action against the hospital staff to prohibit them from administering drugs to him by force in the absence of any emergency. However, the court delineated four factors that must be considered in determining whether an injunction should be issued when a patient refuses medication. These factors are: (1) the patient's capacity to decide on his particular treatment, (2) the patient's physical threat to other patients and to staff at the institution, (3) whether any less restrictive treatments exist, and (4) the risk of permanent side effects from the proposed treatment.

The court held that an involuntary mental patient has a right to refuse medication in the absence of an emergency, as a legitimate exercise of his constitutional right to privacy. In the absence of an emergency, some due process hearing is required prior to forced administration of drugs. This decision, by enumerating the factors to be considered in cases when patients refuse treatment, reflects strides by the court toward establishing further civil liberties for involuntary mental patients. This is not a national standard, however, and a clear statement on refusal of treatment remains to be given by the Supreme Court.

There is little doubt that the growth of civil liberties in this sphere will continue. The day may come when persons suspected of mental illness will have the same procedural and substantive protection as those accused of committing a crime.

Families who are considering having their Alzheimer relative committed should consider that state hospitals no longer warehouse patients. There is a duty to provide treatment to the extent that it can be provided. Consideration is also given to removing from state hospitals patients who do not need intensive types of care; such patients are placed in less restrictive environments. Many Alzheimer patients require an intermediate level of care that may be more efficiently provided in such less restrictive environments as nursing homes. Moving patients into the less restrictive alternative is the sensible course of action for the patients, the staff of institutions, and family members.

CRIMINAL ACTS

Alzheimer patients sometimes act in ways that bring them into conflict with criminal authorities. Such actions as wandering the streets and forgetting to wear proper clothing may attract the attention of police and other law enforcement personnel. In the criminal law there is generally a requirement that an individual must demonstrate criminal intent and know that what he is doing is a crime. If he does not know what he is doing then his legal responsibility diminishes. The consideration of intent will not prevent the police from arresting or detaining an Alzheimer patient, however, nor will they reduce the family's need to try to prevent such events from occurring, but they may relieve the family of some of the anxiety that such behavior may generate.

CIVIL WRONGS

Regardless of their mental condition, Alzheimer patients may still be liable for any civil wrongs committed. In the event that an individual with Alzheimer's has an automobile accident, for example, the owner of the car and the patient could be liable for damages. If the family lives in an apartment and the patient lets a sink overflow and water damages adjoining apartments, both the patient and family may be jointly responsible for the necessary repairs to the other domiciles. The family should give serious consideration to limiting the freedom of an Alzheimer patient when, because of the disease, the risks he poses to himself or others are considerable.

When an Alzheimer's diagnosis is confirmed, the family should include among its various considerations a review of insurance policies to be certain that problems directly traceable to the disease are covered. This review should include both policies covering the home and any automobiles on the premises. Generally, homeowner's insurance provides the most comprehensive type of coverage. An insurance agent familiar with the problems posed by Alzheimer patients would be a good resource for such a review. An Alzheimer support group could also provide the names of a people who might be knowledgeable in this area.

FINDING AN ATTORNEY

When the family needs an attorney to help draft a will, pursue involuntary civil commitment, or secure guardianship of an incapacitated family member, locating a member of the bar who is familiar with this area of the law may present some problems. If there is an Alzheimer support group in the community, members may provide a list of attorneys familiar with the issues and who are experienced. If no support group exists, then a call to the mental health association or the local bar association may prove valuable for those needing a referral list of attorneys specializing in family or mental health law. You are buying a service; do not hesitate to shop around to find an attorney who will work easily with you and your family. A scheduled appointment with several attorneys on the list will be of great help in finding the lawyer best suited to your family's needs.

CONCLUSION

This chapter reviewed guardianship, wills, civil commitment, and other legal matters related to Alzheimer patients. However, there is no substitute for competent legal advice. Each state has its own laws on these matters and the circumstances of each patient and family are unique. I encourage each family to obtain and utilize the services of an attorney familiar with this area of the law. In the long run, many problems can be avoided or their consequences reduced by the use of competent counsel. The earlier the family engages a competent attorney to prepare for the needs of aging individuals, the more time, money, and anxiety will be saved.

Whether or not Alzheimer's disease is present, families should prepare for the care of aging family members, but concern about the illness and incapacity of aging family members is not enough; we must also care enough about ourselves to draft a will and make plans in the event that we become ill or incapacitated. Sometimes the best way to care for others is to care for ourselves.

SUGGESTED READINGS

Cranford, E. R., and Ashley, B. Z. "Ethical and Legal Aspects of Dementia." In *Neurologic Clinics: Dementia,* vol. 4, edited by J. T. Hutton. Philadelphia: W. B. Saunders Company, 1986.

Halleck, S. *Law in the Practice of Psychiatry: A Handbook for Clinicians.* New York: Plenum Medical Book Company, 1980

Hasko, J., Holoch, A., and Young, N. "Gerontology and the Law: A Selected Bibliography." *Southern California Law Review* 289 (1982).

Lieberson, A. D. *The Physician's Guide to Advance Medical Directives.* Los Angeles: PMIC, 1993.

President's Commission for the Study of Ethical Problems in Medicine and Biomedical and Behavioral Research. *Deciding to Forego Life-Sustaining Treatment.* Washington, D.C.: U.S. Government Printing Office, 1983.

16

Ethical Considerations

Thomas F. McGovern

This chapter brings to mind the story of a woman who was being examined in court for possible jury duty. She looked up at the judge and said, "I am sorry, your honor, I can't serve on the jury. I don't believe in capital punishment."

"Maybe you don't understand," the judge said, "this is a civil suit brought by a wife to recover $5,000 of her money spent by her husband on gambling and other women."

"Oh," she said, "I'll serve on the jury, and I could be wrong about capital punishment!"

This humorous story points out that ethical convictions may vary with respect to individuals and the specific circumstances. Most people, however, hold to prevailing ethical principles that assist them in making decisions.

This chapter addresses the ethical considerations which ungird the humane meanings of persons with Alzheimer's. Such considerations challenge our society to support adequately families and health care personnel devoted to the care of persons with the disease. Individual, institutional, and societal values coalesce in developing an ethical response to the human dimensions of Alzheimer's. Here Thomas F. McGovern, an ethicist with a background in counseling and theology, describes a framework for ethical decision making with regard to the care of a person with Alzheimer's disease.

The right to self-determination while one is competent and the right to humane care throughout the course of the disease are of vital interest to

193

victims of Alzheimer's disease, their families, and their caregivers. The principle of justice, too, is of great importance because it calls for the fair treatment of persons experiencing the disease. Ethical values must provide a theoretical and practical basis for social attitudes, which espouse the essential well-being of persons whose ability to care for themselves tragically declines as the disease progresses.

The ethical issues that pertain to the care of persons with Alzheimer's disease embrace at least three broad areas of concern. The first addresses the willingness of our society to provide adequate health care for Alzheimer patients. The second area of concern deals with the right of such persons to direct their lives while they are competent and to have their expressed wishes respected when they become incompetent. The third area of concern focuses on the ethical principles that guide families, caregivers, and institutions as they care for the Alzheimer patient throughout the progressive stages of the disease.

SOCIETAL ATTITUDES

A report of the Presidential Commission for the Study of Ethical Problems in Medicine, *Seeking Access to Health Care* (1983), notes:

> The depth of a society's concern about health care can be seen as a measure of its solidarity in the face of suffering and death. A society's commitment to health care reflects some of its most basic attitudes about what it means to be a member of the human community.

Our society needs to determine the level of health care that will assure both persons with Alzheimer's disease and their families that we truly value them as members of the community. Our present commitment to the health care needs of Alzheimer families is growing but still falls short of what is needed. Recent studies indicate that families provide most of the services needed by Alzheimer patients. The families interviewed indicated that they must exhaust most of their personal resources in order to qualify for Medicaid coverage. The burden they bear can be gauged from the cost of covering four million persons with Alzheimer's in nursing home settings, at an average cost of $60,000 per year (1995 figures).

Those who argue for a right to health care for citizens in general, and in particular for the victims of catastrophic diseases like Alzheimer's, are aware that as a society we tend to limit such rights. It is more realistic to seek an adequate level of health care for persons with Alzheimer's rather than advocate services based on the idea of strict equality in health care. Many find claims based on strict equality to be unacceptable, but they might accept the right to an adequate level, which would guarantee the dignity and self-respect of persons with the disease. In addition, humane and worthy surroundings for care would be provided under such a standard. The details of specific levels of care and a description of humane surroundings would need to be developed to form responsible societal attitudes.

THE PERSON WITH ALZHEIMER'S DISEASE

It is important that the dignity of persons in the early stages of Alzheimer's disease be maintained by involving them in the decision-making process that addresses their present and future welfare. As long as Alzheimer patients retain their decision-making capabilities, they should be encouraged to make a great many personal decisions involving day-to-day living. In addition, provision can be made for the future when persons with Alzheimer's will be unable to make rational decisions. The delicate task of determining present wishes concerning future health care, participation in research, the choice of a nursing home, and the manner of care as death approaches ideally needs to be addressed while the person retains competency. Many of the ethical dilemmas faced by families and caregivers regarding the care of persons in the later stages of the disease could have been anticipated if the patient's wishes had been determined prior to the onset of incompetency. If one waits for such discussions to take place after Alzheimer's disease has been diagnosed, the patient may not be able to comprehend fully the questions at hand. Patients may be totally unaware of their cognitive decline. A lack of awareness makes decision making about unrecognized likelihoods quite problematic. It is perhaps more realistic for such concerns to be discussed prior to the onset of any catastrophic illness.

The involvement of the person with Alzheimer's in making decisions concerning future care is an undertaking that requires tact and sensitivity. Making provisions for the future should not deprive a person of the hope needed for day-to-day living. One must recognize the prevailing reluctance of our society to discuss the types of care or medical interventions we would desire in the final stages of our lives. A contemporary desire for a sudden and anticipated demise is often thwarted by modern medical technology, the advent of which forces us to analyze the essentials of a good death and to embrace the "ars moriendi" (art of dying) wisdom of earlier centuries. In other terminal illnesses, such as cancer, the competent person can make treatment choices throughout the progression of the disease. Those with advanced Alzheimer's disease lack the ability to give such directions. It seems appropriate that a mentally competent adult should determine the essentials of humane care in the later stages of the disease, including specific directions with respect to measures appropriate as death approaches. The desirability or undesirability of heroic measures can be determined by the competent person.

Specific directions about food and fluids often determine when and if artificial feeding is introduced. It would seem appropriate that basic natural satisfactions like eating and drinking should be maintained to the very end for the person with Alzheimer's disease. Human dignity is best preserved through self-feeding or hand-feeding by another. The introduction of tube-feeding can sometimes be the ultimate indignity inflicted on demented persons who have no essential need for it. Understaffed institutions may introduce such procedures in the interest of cost effectiveness and because it is covered by insurance as a part of skilled nursing care. Thoughtful though painful reflection by Alzheimer patients and their caregivers on what constitutes humane care in the later stages of the disease may rescue many a victim from technical forms of care, and assure that compassion will be the primary concern.

Long-term care institutions play a critical role in the provision of humane care for many persons with advanced Alzheimer's disease. Persons in the early stages of the disease are very often able to determine their own futures. Official power of attorney may provide legal assurances that their wishes will be respected (see chapter 15). Family members may struggle to respect the wishes of their loved ones; nursing homes, however, determine if such provisions are realized. It is essential to involve competent persons in the selection of health care facilities that will guarantee humane surroundings, humane care, and respect for the patient's expressed wishes. The presence of a Code of Ethics within the institution and the availability of policies and guidelines with respect to clinical decision making are important considerations in choosing an appropriate facility (see chapter 14). Assurances that the final stages of one's life will be spent in humane surroundings could add immeasurably to the quality of life enjoyed by a person in the early stages of the disease.

The involvement of Alzheimer patients in research activities has attracted most of the recent ethical discussion. The ability of persons in the early or middle stages of the disease to make informed decisions concerning their participation in research is upheld by many ethicists, gerontologists, and legal experts. The present ability of persons with the disease to acquire, retain, process, and act on research information that is appropriately communicated becomes central to the notion of informed consent. It would also seem appropriate that competent persons could consent to continuing in research situations during and after the onset of incompetency. Guarantees should exist, however, that the actual research procedures would not violate individual dignity, expose the person to unnecessary risks, or greatly distress the patient. Institutional Review Boards for the Protection of Human Subjects (IRBs), or their equivalents in nursing home situations, should ensure that adequate protection is afforded persons involved in research and that adequate policies and guidelines spell out this responsibility. Research into the nature of the disease is important, and progress in caring for and treating persons with Alzheimer's is intimately linked to research. Progress, however, is an optional goal and is not worth achieving if individual worth is the price that must be paid. Researchers have an awesome ethical responsibility in assuring that their attitudes reflect respect for the personhood of demented people.

The decision making carried out by persons in the earlier stages of the disease occurs in a familial setting. The decisions made by the persons with the disease are often shaped by the advice of family, friends, and health care professionals. The range of options available to Alzheimer victims is often defined by the ability and willingness of family members and health care professionals to discuss the options and to implement whatever is decided. Meaningful dialogue concerning present and future care is both challenging and rewarding for the patient and the caregiver during the early and middle stages of the disease. It calls for the exercise of ethics in its highest human form because it represents the application of the highest values to the care of human beings.

A caregiver has suggested that a meaningful religious ritual could mark the passage of a person from the semicompetent stage to the demented stage, from the home to the nursing home. Such a ritual would express a belief in the dignity of the person, would give thanks for the blessings of the person's life with special reference to the meaningful times enjoyed since the onset of the disease, and would contain a commitment to the care of the person in the new surroundings. The involvement of competent persons with family and caregivers in planning such life transition rituals could give meaning to an event that is often surrounded by guilt and other negative feelings. Perhaps such a ritual could focus attention on the duties and obligations most appropriate to the care of the persons in the later stages of the disease. In embracing the pain of such decision-making, we might learn the deeper meaning of our service.

ETHICAL ISSUES AND THE CAREGIVER

The family and the health care professional involved in the care of the person with Alzheimer's disease encounter many daily situations in which they must make ethical decisions. These decisions frequently are difficult and may often involve genuine ethical dilemmas. Discussion of the issues can remove some of the perplexity and at the same time illustrate the underlying values, together with practical courses of action that are most appropriate in the care of a person with Alzheimer's disease.

Respect for the person's right to self-determination is the best guarantor of maintaining personal dignity in the early stages of Alzheimer's disease. The ability and the right of such a person to participate in decisions pertaining to present and future care have been presented in the previous section. The willingness of family and health care professionals to guarantee such a right, while assessing and evaluating the person's declining cognitive abilities as the disease progresses, is a difficult task. The advent of incompetence, realizing that a precise definition of such a state does not exist, raises many ethical questions for the caregivers.

The ethical wisdom derived from ongoing discussion about the values and principles that should direct the care of the seriously ill incompetent person is difficult to apply in practice to caregiving situations. Much of the legal and ethical discussion, which often centers on the extreme and ambiguous cases of controversial medical decision making, has an academic flavor that seems incongruent with the human anguish that occurs as a result of such difficult decisions. A humane understanding of the issues necessarily includes an analysis of the ethical and legal principles involved; but it must also include descriptions of how these principles are translated into humane care. George Bateson writes that in the attainment of grace, the reasons of the heart must be integrated with the reason of the reason. A purely rational, intellectual, and ethical approach to the needs of the person with Alzheimer's disease will not work of itself; neither will a purely emotional approach.

The attitudes of caregivers toward caring for persons with advanced dementing disease are determined in part by the caregivers' views of the personhood of the demented individual. For many caregivers, caring for the body of the Alzheimer patient often stands as a metaphor for taking care of the mind and the spirit of the whole person. For these individuals an essential value is acknowledged by providing even the most basic care for victims of this disease. Another approach that might be espoused by caregivers would emphasize the loss of personhood, identity, and self-reflection by the person with Alzheimer's disease. Advocates of this position argue that to recognize the diminished personhood of the patient reduces guilt and frustration in the family and in caregivers, which ultimately results in reduced stress and, paradoxically, produces more effective care. Viewing victims of Alzheimer's disease as less than persons, however, can quickly lead to their total devaluation as nonpersons. The status of nonperson is perilous because such a being does not enjoy the privileges and rights of human beings and, as such, is easily discounted.

The value system of the caregiver serves as the ultimate basis for the care provided to the Alzheimer patient. The ethical perspectives of caregivers determine in real life their reactions to routine and emergency situations. The manner in which a caregiver defines a "problem" will determine the clinical interventions. A person's beliefs about the patient, the disease, and dying will often decide the treatment or procedure that is instituted. The desirability of tube feeding as opposed to the trouble of more normal feeding is strongly influenced by the value system of the caregiver and of the institution. The dignity of the dying person is best assured by caregivers who know how to comfort such patients. This calls for skill, compassion, honesty, and humility. The practical application of compassion is a powerful determinant of the quality of care enjoyed by those patients experiencing the later stages of the disease and, ultimately, in their final act of dying.

Compassion and mercy in caregivers are the qualities that are best suited to meeting the needs of demented persons in all phases of their disease. Little has been written about the practical application of such qualities to the care of the seriously ill. Scant attention is paid to these concepts in the training of health care professionals. The overwhelming emphasis in professional schools is on the technical aspects of patient care. Caring for the demented person in the late and final stages of illness is a high human and professional calling that fully challenges the art and science of the caregiver. Mind and heart are wedded in the care of critically ill demented persons whose most basic human satisfaction may be derived from such basic activities as sucking on a thumb. The sounds, the touch, the smells, the food, the drink, the sensory stimulation that comfort or give pleasure to the severely demented are the human components that constitute the practice of mercy and compassion in the care of persons undergoing the late and final stages of Alzheimer's disease. The human qualities that enable caregivers to deliver such care merit serious attention. People who are comfortable with the unusual, who have basic physical, emotional, and spiritual resilience together with warmth and a sense of humor, may be best suited for the challenging role of caregiver. Those who provide care create the human environment in which concern, fairness, compassion, and mercy translate into effective, humane care for persons in the later and final stages of Alzheimer's disease.

The development of a Code of Ethics to guide families and caregivers in the application of ethical principles to the care of persons in advanced stages of the disease would be helpful. Policies and guidelines covering many issues of care could be drawn from such a code. Ethics committees would also be a welcome addition because of their ability to provide education, consultation, and case review in difficult decision-making situations. Some have expressed concern about the quality of the decision making that occurs in nursing homes, which are sometimes described as a very troubled and troublesome component of the health care system. The absence of input from physicians and other skilled health care professionals, because of the limited role they play in such institutions, is noted in this respect.

An ethical code, directed toward the specific needs of persons with cancer, has been adopted by M. D. Anderson Hospital in Houston, Texas. The code is intended to give impetus and direction when thinking about moral problems, but it does not attempt to solve them. An impressive statement of institutional concern for the dignity of persons with cancer is found in the use of the term *reverence for the patient* as the essential determinant of the institution's approach. A model code, which would provide similar direction for institutions involved in the care of persons with Alzheimer's disease and for research in the field, could be developed by the Alzheimer's Disease and Related Disorders Association or some other interested group. The moral values of families and caregivers, which undergird the care given to persons with this disease, need to be incorporated into a code that could benefit all who are touched by Alzheimer's disease.

The Alzheimer's Association (1995) has developed commendable guidelines which address the needs of persons with Alzheimer's in long-term care facilities. These guidelines call for the creation of "compassionate life-enriching programs and environments." Likewise, the Ethics Committee of the Alzheimer's Association is developing a code of ethics which addresses issues of human dignity in caring for persons with Alzheimer's.

Reflection on the values that surround the care of a person with Alzheimer's disease can be a rewarding experience for families and caregivers: it highlights their heroic efforts to maintain the dignity of the patients in their care. Discussion of humane care in the later and final stages of the disease helps concerned caregivers identify the essential human elements of such care. Ethical reflection also safeguards the rights of seriously demented persons whose welfare is totally determined by others. As we engage in the pain and suffering of the individuals with the disease, and their families, and seek to care for them in their need, we discover within ourselves depths of concern, compassion, and mercy that remind us of our essential human value.

CONCLUSION

Many reports indicate the existence of major gaps in the care of persons with Alzheimer's disease and in support systems for their families. The gaps occur in: treatment, efforts to assist families of persons with Alzheimer's disease, alternative systems of care, training of research and clinical personnel, educational materials and information dissemination for the public and professionals, and financing systems of care. The essential ethical issue facing our society is the provision of adequate care for those with the disease; the absence of such care can no longer be excused on the basis of a lack of information about the existence and prevalence of Alzheimer's disease. Callahan (1995) argues that the selfhood of persons with Alzheimer's demands that vigorous efforts to promote the most supportive environment be in place until the late stages of the disease. He points to the progress being made in maintaining the cognitive well-being of persons throughout many stages of the disease.

Ambiguity and uncertainty are to be expected in dealing with the issues of care for persons with Alzheimer's disease. Despite such diffi-culties, a humane society can meet the challenge by providing a true com-munity of care in which human dignity is assured throughout the tragic course of the disease. The demise of competency and self-awareness must not be seen as a loss of personhood; the loss of the ability to be self-deter-mining does not rob a person of basic human dignity. A person with Alzheimer's disease remains a human person throughout the course of the disease. To be considered less than human exposes such nonpersons to the danger of being discarded as unworthy of rights and privileges. Our soci-ety has a profound ethical responsibility to respect the Alzheimer patient and to align itself with heroic family members and dedicated health care professionals in providing optimal care for the victims of this disease. Ethical relation, at the individual, institutional, and societal levels, must be an ongoing reality if the well-being of persons with Alzheimer's dis-ease and their families is to be assured.

SUGGESTED READINGS

Alzheimer's Association. *Guidelines for Dignity: Goals of Specialized Alzheim-er/Dementia Care in Residential Settings.* Chicago: Alzheimer's Associa-tion, 1992.

Boyle, J. M. "The Developing Consensus on the Right to Health Care." In *Jus-tice and Health Care,* edited by M. J. Kelly. St. Louis: The Catholic Health Association of the United States, 1984.

Callahan, D. "Terminating Life-Sustaining Treatment of the Demented." *Hast-ings Center Report* 6 (1995): 25–31.

Childress, J. F. "Ensuring Care, Respect, and Fairness for the Elderly." *Hastings Center Report* 14 (1984): 27–31.

Capron, A. M. "Ironies and Tensions in the Feeding of the Dying." *Hastings Cen-ter Report* 14 (1984): 32–35.

Cassell, E. J. "Do Justice, Love Mercy: The Inappropriateness of the Concept of Justice Applied to Bedside Decisions." In *Justice and Health Care,* edited by E. E. Shelp. Boston: D. Reidel Publishing Company, 1981.

———. "Life as a Work of Art." *Hastings Center Report* 14 (1984): 35–37.

Fried, C. "Equality and Rights in Medical Care." *Hastings Center Report* 6 (1976): 29–34.

Gaylin, W. "In Defense of the Dignity of Being Human." *Hastings Center Report* 14 (1984): 18–22.

Glaser, J. W. *Three Realms of Ethics.* Kansas City, Mo.: Sheed and Ward, 1994.

Green, W. "Setting Boundaries for Artificial Feeding." *Hastings Center Report* 14 (1984): 8–10.

Hermann, H. T. "Ethical Dilemmas Intrinsic to the Care of Elderly Demented Patients." *Journal of American Geriatric Society* 32 (1984): 655–56.

Howell, M. "Caretakers' Views on Responsibilities for the Care of the Demented Elderly." *Journal of American Geriatric Society* 32 (1984): 657–60.

Kitwood, T., and Bredin, K. "Toward a Theory of Dementia Care: Personhood and Well-Being." *Aging and Society* 12 (1992): 269–87.

McCormick, R. "Caring or Starving: The Case of Claire Conroy." *America* (April 6, 1985): 269–73.

President's Commission for the Study of Ethical Problems in Medicine and Bio-medical and Behavioral Research. *Deciding to Forego Life-Sustaining Treatment.* Washington, D.C.: U.S. Government Printing Office, 1983.

———. *Securing Access to Health Care,* vol. 1. Washington, D.C.: U.S. Government Printing Office, 1983.

17

Medical Breakthroughs: Real or Illusory?

Trudy Hutton and J. Thomas Hutton

Progress in the diagnosis and treatment of Alzheimer's disease has made painfully slow yet steady progress in the last decade. With the devastating toll Alzheimer's wreaks on the nearly 4 million victims in the United States and their families, at an estimated cost of $100 billion per year, it is little wonder that patients and families seek information on every modicum of progress in the battle against Alzheimer's disease. Announcements of new discoveries appear regularly in the popular press, often arousing an excitement that cools as the initial reports appear overstated.

In the last decade the popular press has regularly reported "breakthroughs" in the diagnosis and treatment of Alzheimer's disease, frequently with sensational headlines and stories. "NEW HOPE FOR ALZHEIMER'S VICTIMS" was the headline beckoning from the June 18, 1990, issue of *Time* magazine. The article reported that "it will soon be easier to identify Alzheimer's earlier and more accurately" and went on to claim that "Alzheimer's appears to be yielding to treatment." Reports in the intervening years have proven the tests and treatment discussed in the *Time* article to be less than the headlines indicated. The statement that "it will soon be easier to identify Alzheimer's earlier and more accurately" stemmed from an article in the *Journal of the American Medical Association* that described a biochemical test capable of correctly identifying 86 percent of brain samples of Alzheimer sufferers taken at autopsy. The article reported that scientists expected within two years to develop a test to detect the Alzheimer disease-associated protein in the spinal fluid, hence giving rise to an effective clinical diagnostic tool. The second statement, that "Alzheimer's appears to be yielding to treatment," resulted from an application to the Food and Drug Administration by the Warner-Lambert pharmaceutical firm to market a drug called Cognex, the brand name for tacrine, also referred to as THA (tetrahydroaminoacridine). The article reported that the drug "supposedly slows the loss of brain function in 40 percent of Alzheimer's patients who are given the medication and could conceivably add one or more productive years to the lives of Alzheimer's victims."

Four years later *Newsweek* reported "tacrine hydrochloride is of limited usefulness and only in the early stages of the disease" (November 21, 1994). In the fall of 1996 *Time* recounted that "while some patients who take tacrine benefit from subtle to moderate improvements in mood and short-term memory, many others do not. Moreover, tacrine can produce a raft of side effects" (Fall 1996). The test using spinal fluid is not yet the diagnostic tool predicted in 1990 and its results and application are still being examined; yet is has recently been touted once again as a "new diagnostic tool" (*U.S. News and World Report,* April 8, 1996). News reports in 1994 heralded: "There's still no cure in sight, but a new test, using eye drops, could be a breakthrough" (*Newsweek,* November 21, 1994). The article described how the eye drops caused the pupils of Alzheimer's patients to dilate approximately four times as much as normal controls. Nineteen ninety-five brought announcements of the discovery of more "new genes thought to be responsible for Alzheimer's disease" and in 1996 the "possible antidotes to Alzheimer's" were reported to be estrogen and aspirin (*U.S. News and World Report,* August 26, 1996 and September 16, 1996). *Newsweek* and *Science News* recounted in 1996 that Alzheimer's disease may soon be predicted through brain scans and changes in writing samples.

Such articles tantalize readers, but are these claims of medical breakthroughs real or illusory? The reporting in these news articles was no better or worse than the many others published, but they can be used to illustrate the difference between medical advancements and the much-hoped-for breakthroughs in finding the cause(s) of, effective treatment(s) for, and potential cure(s) for Alzheimer's disease. Interpreting such announcements with a critical eye can reduce unrealistic public expectations and still allow hope for the future.

WHAT IS A BREAKTHROUGH?

It is helpful to characterize and compare what is meant by a breakthrough, first for the scientist and then for the family caregiver. The scientist views breakthroughs as major advances in the understanding of a disease. For example, understanding that an abnormal protein exists in the brain tissue of Alzheimer victims, that a genetic anomaly exists on a chromosome or chromosomes, or that the principal biochemical abnormality in Alzheimer brain tissue is a deficiency of the chemical acetylcholine represent fundamental improvements in scientific understanding. How a person's pupils react to eye drops or how one's handwriting changes are small but potentially significant pieces to the puzzle that is Alzheimer's disease. The scientist uses small bits of newly uncovered information to study, interpret, and apply these data to other theories, perhaps his own or those of a colleague, hoping to discover other parts to the puzzle. Eventually the scientific community seeks to reveal a more complete understanding of the disease. Repetitions of an experiment or study help to confirm or refute a certain theory or a given treatment. Demonstrating that an experiment or treatment is negative may have as much significance for a researcher as a positive outcome. Small theoretical advances may be of utmost importance for the scientist even though their therapeutic value is years away. These small victories may prove to be real "breakthroughs" in the laboratory.

Such information, however, does not immediately lead to improvements in the day-to-day care of afflicted persons, nor does it identify the cause or suggest a cure for the disorder. To family caregivers, such improvements in knowledge may seem trivial. To concerned family members, only an effective treatment or a means to slow the inexorable slide to severe dementia could be a real "breakthrough." Because the media coverage of current medical research into various diseases is open to interpretation, readers of research articles or those who hear a dramatic news release must scrutinize the claims critically.

The tacrine story is a perfect example of the danger of overemphasizing much-touted reports in scientific as well as popular publications that claim amazing benefits for some new treatment. Despite widespread criticism of the original THA study for being faulty in its methods, publication of the results led to considerable pressure to treat Alzheimer patients with tacrine. Such reactions to preliminary and unreplicated results of a treatment are understandable but should be tempered by putting the new research into proper perspective. Six years later tacrine is widely considered to provide only a modest and temporary respite to the ravages of Alzheimer's. Important new studies that sound hopeful but later prove to be unfounded may result not only in raising unrealistic expectations among patients and family members but also in developing potentially risky treatments that have little or no positive effect.

ANALYZING ANNOUNCEMENTS

When announcements of a new treatment or a new "breakthrough" appear in the media, readers/listeners must take care to analyze them in order to properly assess the claims being made and to sort the pertinent information from the extraneous verbiage used to catch consumer attention. Several points should be kept in mind to avoid false expectations on the part of patients and family members.

First, one must not be misled by headlines that are created to call attention to a story. Words used in headlines are specifically calculated to heighten consumer interest. In the *Time* magazine article, "New Hope for Alzheimer's Victims," the wording was selected to entice those with any interest in the disease to spend the time to read what this "new hope" was. More recent articles may not have the sensational wording, but still entice readers to read farther. "Estrogen cuts risk of Alzheimer's" (*Science News,* September 7, 1996) and ". . . a new test, using eye drops, could be a breakthrough" (*Newsweek,* November 4, 1994) put a spin on the headlines and lead paragraph that encourages high and hopeful expectations if the articles are not analyzed with a critical eye.

In both popular articles and scientific reports, readers should take special note of all disclaimers and qualifiers used to describe a "breakthrough" or the new finding being disclosed. The *Time* article was replete with such disclaimers and qualifiers; for example, the article stated that: "Alzheimer's finally *appears* to be *yielding* to treatment"; "a new biochemical test . . . *may* prove to be highly reliable in detecting a collection of molecules . . . found only in patients with the illness"; scientists *expect* . . . to develop a test (to detect Alzheimer's disease from spinal fluid)"; ". . . tacrine, a drug that *supposedly slows* the loss of brain function . . ."; and ". . . *could conceivably* add one or more productive years to the lives of Alzheimer's victims." The *Newsweek* article describing the eye drop test stated that this was ". . . the first simple and *apparently* accurate test for the disease . . ." *U.S. News and World Reports* stated that ". . . aspirin and other . . . nonsteroidal anti-inflammatory drugs, *used regularly may* reduce in the *risk* of mental decline in old age by 20 percent." The importance of such qualifiers is frequently overlooked by Alzheimer sufferers and family members who are grasping for any sign of hope, for some positive information in their search for effective treatment and cure. Estrogen, according to *U.S. News and World Reports*, "*could* lower [the] *risk* of developing Alzheimer's," but went on to qualify the article by stating that because of possible side effects, researchers still had reservations about the use of estrogen to prevent Alzheimer's.

In addition to paying close attention to the manner in which a story is worded, readers/listeners should also consider the source of the story. The veracity of the source should be considered: Is the news source known for accurate and competent reporting or does it have a reputation for sensationalizing stories in order to gain attention? Evaluate, if possible, the source of the news article. Is the story from a national news service or the result of local reporting? Is it paraphrased from the original source? Try to determine if the person presenting the results is an expert in the field, with firsthand knowledge of the story, or if the report is a summary of a more detailed paper written by someone else. Analyze whether the reporter specializes in reporting medical news or is someone who reports general topics. Consumers can call or write the news source and ask for more details concerning the reports they choose to analyze.

If possible, find out where the information was reported or originated. Try to determine if it is the result of a controlled study in a major medical center specializing in the particular research area or if it is an isolated report from a small group or from a single investigator. The background of the investigator reporting the results may be significant: Is this person someone who specializes in the area and has done previous work on the subject, or is the researcher new to the field? Ascertain the person's experience and standing among professional peers. Although some breakthroughs may certainly come from a small medical center recently embarking on research in a particular area, chances are that major findings would come from research centers with a history of competent work that investigates the subject.

Examine the procedure utilized to obtain the results reported. Ask if the particular report discusses an original study or describes a replication of some previous study. Look at the number of patients participating, the length of the study, and whether it was an open study or a blinded one.* Consider if the study has been reported in the scientific literature prior to publication in the popular press. If the material has appeared in the scientific literature, ask if the particular publication in which it appeared is "peer reviewed," that is, whether other competent scientists in the field reviewed and critiqued the material prior to publication.

There may be a delay of many months between the time data are presented at a conference, submitted for publication, and actually published as an article in a scientific journal. During this period, if the information is deemed newsworthy, the popular press may publish a version of the findings. Consider, however, if the findings have been presented to a scientific meeting prior to publication and if the results of the study are available. Frequently the media choose to publicize what they consider to be the most exciting, the most favorable, and the more enthusiastic reports, while ignoring less favorable or negative studies. Enthusiastic reports may make a better story but negative results can be just as important in the study of a particular disease. It is here that the experience and expertise of the reporter may influence the information selected for the news report. The selection of information may determine whether the subsequent report is accurate or results in mistranslating or misunderstanding of the data actually presented.

The news report may be so worded as to create a false impression of what has been presented. This may be done inadvertently, by leaving out important facts and selectively reporting those that seem to be most exciting, or it may be done in order to catch the listener's attention. In either instance, a false impression can be created.

Judge the slant given to the news report. Look for comments on the particular study from experts and consider if the various experts have been quoted at length or if the quotes have been severely edited such that the report is given a certain slant or bias making it sound more favorable and thus more exciting as a news report. Uncritical media reports may lead to confusion; they sometimes create a false public impression of what has actually been demonstrated.

---

*In an open study, both the patient and the investigator know if the patient is taking an active agent (the drug being tested) or a placebo (an inactive agent) during the trial period. This type of study lends itself to more subjective interpretation of a test than does a blinded study. In a single-blind study, the investigator knows whether a patient is taking a placebo or active drug, but the patient does not know which he is taking. In a double-blind study, neither the investigator nor the patient knows which kind of agent (study drug) the patient is taking. Blinded studies are given much more weight since there is less opportunity for scientific bias.

When analyzing a report of some scientific finding, it is important to consider personal biases toward the subject. Do readers/listeners *want* to perceive the report as more favorable than it actually is? Do readers/listeners selectively retain only what is wanted: those bits of information that are positive and perhaps offer more hope than some others? In selectively retaining portions of the material presented, they may create in their own minds false expectations and thereby mistranslate what is in fact said.

Once readers/listeners have analyzed the validity of the report, they must assess the impact of the information. For example, if a new drug treatment is reported, they should look for its availability to the general public. Is the drug still in an experimental stage? Is the report preliminary or a long-term summary? Has the drug been tested long enough to determine its side effects? Determine if the drug is or soon will be available to the public and, if so, how readily available it is (will be). If the treatment is not available, inquire as to whether application for marketing has been made. When such reports reach the popular press, interested persons should ask their doctors about the drug: family physicians or internists may have knowledge of the study discussed, and in any case they are good sources of information. Frequently doctors have access to the original report or to relevant data and are able to interpret the results more accurately.

Recently another source of information for Alzheimer research has burst on the scene and the information available multiplies daily. The Internet has become easily accessible to the general public as a source of an immense body of information. The Internet is a vast computer network allowing virtually anyone with a home computer and the proper software to obtain information from anywhere in the world. Not only does one have access to information published in the popular press, but also to scientific publications and reports.

The Internet had its beginnings when the Defense Department decided that it would be efficient for researchers in their large national laboratories and universities to be able to communicate among their computer networks. In the last several years the number of people connected to the Internet has virtually exploded. No longer is this communication network used only by researchers working on commercial computer systems. Elementary school students and retirees alike are taking advantage of the incredible amounts of information available on the Internet. Not only is one able to access books and magazines published in the United

States through the Library of Congress, but also virtually any major university library in the world. In addition to access to published materials, Internet users can talk to one another. Through the amazing technology of e-mail, one can ask and respond to questions and comments from the immense number of e-mail users. Everything from recipes to treatments for disease and comparisons of medications is discussed via the Internet, and this is where one must also be critical in analyzing the information received.

THE PROCESS OF DRUG RESEARCH

Upon hearing reports of new treatments, we must realize and appreciate the long, slow research process involved from the stage of initial theory to the actual public availability of any therapy. Many potential compounds have been proposed but the vast majority fall by the wayside at some stage of the approval process.

The research to develop a treatment for Alzheimer's disease, or any other disorder, is a slow process at best. It has been estimated that about ten years are required from the time of initial research to the availability of a new medicine for public use. Approximately five of every four thousand compounds screened are approved for human testing, and of those five only one is approved for physicians to prescribe to their patients. Research begins with a body of theoretical knowledge that must be applied to the problem presented. The development of new treatments begins with basic laboratory research. This research is funded by grants from the government, private agencies, and pharmaceutical companies.

Preclinical testing begins with basic pharmacology and animal trials. These tests show how the disease may affect the body and how a compound may work against that effect. The basic research also determines how the compound behaves in the body, what its characteristics are, any toxicity caused by the compound, and evidence of safety for further usage. This stage usually lasts one to two years. At this point the sponsoring company usually files an application for an Investigational New Drug (IND) with the Food and Drug Administration. The application must show, among other things, the results of all experiments to date, the drug's chemical makeup, how it works in the body, any toxic effects, and any research that has been published on similar compounds anywhere in the world. Once the FDA has approved an IND application, the drug can be tested on human subjects.

Three phases exist in the human testing stage of any drug. After each phase, the sponsor must apply to proceed with the next step. The sponsor must submit and have approved a protocol of the planned test. This protocol specifies the methods proposed to administer the drug, the description of the specific tests, the criteria for selecting subjects who will be allowed to participate, and the extensive laboratory tests that will be required to monitor them.

Phase I involves testing of the drug on a small number of volunteers, usually healthy subjects, for a fairly short period of time. This phase helps delineate such things as how the drug acts on the body, safe dosage ranges, side effects, and the duration of the drug's effectiveness. Phase I testing lasts about one year.

Phase II testing consists of controlled studies in larger numbers of volunteer patients, that is, people who have the disease. The Phase II tests are usually limited to a small number of patients for a short period of time. The total clinical testing period for this phase, however, is about two years. Extensive laboratory tests are required to monitor the effect of the drug on the patients and to identify any adverse reactions. This phase of testing is usually conducted at several facilities by various teams of investigators. The facilities and investigators must receive approval by the FDA as well as approval from their own institution to participate.

Phase III consists of testing, on even larger numbers of volunteer patients under conditions similar to those existing in ordinary medical practice. Physicians who are expert in dealing with the condition for which the drug is being tested are invited to participate. Patients are monitored over a longer period of time to detect the effect of the medication on the disease as well as any side effects caused by the longer-term usage. This phase usually lasts approximately three years.

During these phases of testing, the investigators must maintain careful clinical records for all patients participating in the study and report all effects of the medication, both positive and negative. These records are subject to periodic audits by FDA representatives.

Reports of the clinical experiments with new drugs are presented at scientific meetings by the various investigators. Frequently, it is at such meetings that the popular press hears and reports on what has been presented. Through such accounts, patients and their families hear about potential treatments. This often puts pressure on the investigators to make the drug(s) available. However, it may be some time before the drug is widely available for prescription.

Once all three phases of clinical trials have been completed, the sponsor of the drug must go before the FDA with a New Drug Application (NDA) containing all of the information that has been gathered on the drug, its chemical structure, the results of all of the testing on both animals and humans, as well as how the sponsor proposes to manufacture and label the drug for general use. Review of the NDA takes approximately two to three years. After all of the material has been reviewed, only one in five drugs approved for human testing is subsequently approved for marketing to the general public.

Even after a medication is available for physicians to prescribe for their patients, sponsoring companies must continue to submit evaluations of the drug's long-term effects. After FDA approval, companies must do large-scale manufacturing and distribution of the drug as well as physician education about its usage. The cost of developing a single new medicine can be as much as $200 million.

Despite the long, complicated, and expensive procedures involved in developing new drugs, the future holds much promise for Alzheimer's patients and their families. As indicated by the media attention to the disease, advancement in research is not only in the forefront of the news but a goal of laboratories throughout the country. There are many talented scientists and clinical investigators studying all aspects of Alzheimer's disease from physiological changes in the body to new drugs that may lead to more effective treatment. As of March 1996, fourteen pharmaceutical companies were testing sixteen new drugs for the treatment of Alzheimer's disease. In addition to these new agents in various phases of testing, researchers are also investigating the potential of using existing drugs in the treatment of Alzheimer's disease. How such drugs as estrogen supplements, antioxidants such as vitamin E, and aspirin and other anti-inflammatory drugs will effect the development and course of Alzheimer's disease remains to be seen.

One of these studies may lead to the "breakthrough" scientists need to pursue their research into the cause of the disease. One of them may result in the "breakthrough" that patients and families are seeking for effective treatment, maybe even a cure for Alzheimer's disease. Until that time, each person should learn as much as possible about the disease while critically analyzing information provided in media reports. Careful analysis of these reports on current research will enable Alzheimer sufferers and their families to stay abreast of recent advances without indulging in unrealistic expectations while at the same time maintaining hope for the future.

ALZHEIMER'S MEDICINES IN DEVELOPMENT

Drugs in Development for Alzheimer's Disease (U.S.)

Drug	Company	Status
AF102B	Forest Laboratories	Phase III
ALCAR (acetyl-l-carnitine)	Sigma-Tau Pharmaceuticals	Phase III
BIIP-20	Boehringer Ingelheim	Phase II
DHEA (dihydroepiandrosterone)	Neurocrine Biosciences	Phase II
E2020	Eisai; Pfizer	Phase III
eptastigmine (MF-201)	Mediolanum Pharmaceuticals	Phase II
Milameline	Warner Lambert	Phase III
propentofylline	Hoechst-Roussel Pharmaceuticals	Phase III
Reminyl™ (sabeluzole)	Janssen Pharmaceutical	Phase III
SB202026	SmithKline Beecham	Phase II
SDZ ENA-713	Sandoz Pharmaceuticals	Phase III
Sermion® (nicergoline)	Pharmacia & Upjohn	Phase II
SR 46559	Sanofi	Phase II
SR 57746	Sanofi	Phase II
Synapton (physostigmine)	Forest Laboratories	Phase III
xanomeline (LY 246708)	Eli Lilly	Phase II

Contributors

PAUL K. CHAFETZ, PH.D., is assistant professor of gerontology and geriatric services at the University of Texas Southwestern Medical Center at Dallas. He is the coauthor of "Overcoming Obstacles to Cooperation in Interdisciplinary Long-term Care Teams," *Journal of Gerontological Social Work* (Spring 1988). He also authored "Communicating Effectively with Elderly Clients," *Seminars in Speech and Language* (Spring 1988). His research focuses on special care units for dementia victims in nursing homes. He maintains a private practice in clinical gerontological psychology in Dallas.

ROGER F. CLEM, M.S., CCC-A, CED, was formerly an instructor and clinical supervisor in the Department of Communicative Disorders at the Lamar University Speech and Hearing Center. He was a consultant to the Ministry of Education, Shan Dong Province of the People's Republic of China. He is the author of a paper titled "Tejas-Mainland China's Programs for the Hearing-impaired," which was presented in the Spring of 1987.

MORRIS CRAIG, PH.D., is a long-term care consultant and former director of the Texas Department of Health–Alzheimer's Program. He is the author of "Texas Health Advocacy Services Long-Term Care Network" published by the American Association of Retired Persons (1994), "How to Manage the Alzheimer's Patient: Behavior Problems," published by the Texas Department of Health (1985), and "Alzheimer's and the Legal Profession," published jointly by the Office of the Attorney General of Texas and the Texas

Department of Health (1986). He serves on the Joint Commission of Accreditation of Health Care Organizations–Long-Term Care Professionals Committee, Health and Long-Term Care Committee, National American Association of Retired Persons, Texas Medical Foundation Master Committee, and the Texas Medical Foundation Beneficiary Liaison Committee. He served on the 1995 White House Conference on Aging.

RAYE LYNNE DIPPEL, PH.D., is a clinical and lifespan developmental psychologist. She was formerly an assistant professor in the Department of Psychiatry at the University of Texas Medical School at Houston and in the Department of Psychology at Lamar University in Beaumont, Texas, and is currently in private practice in Colorado Springs, Colorado. Dr. Dippel is co-editor (with J. Thomas Hutton) of *Caring for the Parkinson Patient: A Practical Guide,* Amherst, N.Y.: Prometheus Books (1989).

ROBERT G. HARPER, PH.D., is associate professor of psychology at Baylor College of Medicine in Houston, Texas. He has done joint research and has coauthored articles with Doreen Kotik-Harper on assessment of dependence and cognitive functioning.

J. RAY HAYS, PH.D., J.D., is professor of psychiatry and behavioral science at the University Texas Medical School in Houston. His primary clinical work assignment is at the Harris County Psychiatric Center where he works with many demented patients and their families. Along with Robert Meyer and Rhett Landis, he is the author of *Law for the Psychotherapist,* New York: W. W. Norton and Company (1988).

JANICE R. HERMANN, PH.D., R.D., is assistant professor in the Department of Foods, Nutrition, and Institutional Administration at Oklahoma State University. She is the author of "Healthy Aging: A Community Program for the Older Adult," Oklahoma State University Cooperative Extension Service (1986).

J. THOMAS HUTTON, M.D., PH.D., is in the private practice of neurology and directs the Neurology Research Center at St. Mary of the Plains Hospital in Lubbock, Texas. Previously he was professor of medical and surgical neurology at Texas Tech Alzheimer's Disease Institute. Dr. Hutton also was the founding chairman of the Texas Council on Alzheimer's Disease and Related Disorders. He is co-editor (with A. D. Kenny) of *Senile*

Dementia of the Alzheimer Type, New York: Alan R. Liss, Inc. (1985); editor of *Dementia* (Neurologic Clinics), Philadelphia: W. B. Saunders Co. (1986); and co-editor (with Raye Lynne Dippel) of *Caring for the Parkinson Patient: A Practical Guide,* Amherst, N.Y.: Prometheus Books (1989).

TRUDY HUTTON, J.D., is coordinator of the American Parkinson Disease Association Information and Referral Center in Lubbock, Texas. She also the patient coordinator for the Neurology Research Center at St. Mary the Plains Hospital. As an attorney, she specializes in family law. In addition, Ms. Hutton has long experience in education and working with families of neurological patients.

ESPERANZA V. JOYCE, ED.D., R.N., CNS, is associate professor of family nursing care at Texas A&M University–Corpus Christi.

KENN M. KIRKSEY, PH.D., R.N., CS, CEN, APN, is associate professor of acute nursing care at Texas A&M University–Corpus Christi.

DOREEN KOTIK-HARPER, PH.D., is assistant professor of family practice at the University of Texas Health Sciences Center–Houston, and director of behavioral sciences for the family practice residency program for Memorial Hospital. She has done joint research and has coauthored articles with Robert Harper on assessment of dementia and cognitive functioning.

JOANNE S. LINDOERFER, PH.D., is associate professor of psychology at Lamar University in Beaumont, Texas. She maintains a clinical family-oriented private practice and has assisted the families of many Alzheimer patients.

THOMAS F. MCGOVERN, ED.D., is associate professor of psychiatry in the School of Medicine, Texas Tech University Health Sciences Center in Lubbock. He has given many lectures and has written numerous articles on ethical issues in caring for the aged, drug dependency in the elderly, as well as loss and grief. He has developed an active research program that focuses on understanding the memory difficulties of Alzheimer patients.

DAVID B. MITCHELL, PH.D., is associate professor of psychology at Loyola University in Chicago, Illinois. He is coauthor (with R. R. Hunt and

F. A. Schmitt) of "The Generation Effect and Reality Monitoring: Evidence from Dementia and Normal Aging," *Journal of Gerontology* (1986), and "Implicit and Explicit Memory for Pictures: Multiple Views Across the Lifespan," in *Implicit Memory: New Directions in Cognition, Development, and Neuropsychology*, Hillsdale, N.J.: Erlbaum (1993).

JERRY L. MORRIS, M.A., is a research associate at the Neurology Research and Education Center at St. Mary of the Plains in Lubbock, Texas.

VIRGINIA A. SEELBACH, M.ED., was a program specialist for the Southeast Texas Area Agency for Aging in Nederland, Texas, and has presented many papers on the needs of Alzheimer families.

WAYNE C. SEELBACH, PH.D., is Vice President of Academic Affairs and the Provost of Montevello University in Birmingham, Alabama. He is the author of "Filial Responsibility and the Care of Aging Family Members," in *Independent Aging: Family and Social Systems Perspectives*, Rockville, Md.: Aspen System Corporation (1984).

JOYCE E. SHAHEEN, PH.D., was formerly an assistant professor of psychology at Lamar University in Beaumont, Texas. She is a member of the Gerontological Society and frequently lectures and gives seminars on aging.

JO ANN SHROYER, PH.D., is assistant professor in the Department of Merchandising, Environmental Design, and Consumer Economics at Texas Tech University in Lubbock. She is the author of "Alzheimer Patient: Interior Design Considerations," *Texas Medicine* (1987), and "Alzheimer Disease Victims: Behavior-environmental Relationship," *Southwestern Journal of Aging* (1987).

BEVERLY SMYTHIA, B.S., is the founder and former president of the Greater Beaumont (Texas) Chapter of the Alzheimer's Association. She is currently a board member of that organization and a member of the Alzheimer's Association Coalition Chapter of Texas. She is a special education teacher at Lumberton Middle School and mother to three teenagers.

JULIAN E. SPALLHOLZ, PH.D., is professor of nutrition and director of the Institute for Nutritional Sciences at Texas Tech University in Lubbock.

He is coauthor of "Association of Minerals and Metabolic Imbalances with Alzheimer's and Other Dementias," *Texas Medicine* (1987).

BERRY N. SQUYRES, M.D. (deceased), was professor emeritus of family medicine at the Texas Tech University Health Sciences Center in Lubbock. He was director of the Medical Student Clerkship and former chairman of the Department of Family Medicine (1978–1986).